Cardiovascular Review

Guest Editor

BOBBI LEEPER, MN, RN, CNS, CCRN, FAHA

CRITICAL CARE NURSING CLINICS OF NORTH AMERICA

www.ccnursing.theclinics.com

Consulting Editor
JANET FOSTER, PhD, RN, CNS

December 2011 • Volume 23 • Number 4

SAUNDERS an imprint of ELSEVIER, Inc.

W.B. SAUNDERS COMPANY
A Division of Elsevier Inc.

Elsevier Inc., 1600 John F. Kennedy Blvd., Suite 1800, Philadelphia, PA 19103-2899

http://www.theclinics.com

CRITICAL CARE NURSING CLINICS OF NORTH AMERICA Volume 23, Number 4
December 2011 ISSN 0899-5885, ISBN-13: 978-1-4557-0665-5

Editor: Katie Hartner
Developmental Editor: Donald E. Mumford

Critical Care Nursing Clinics of North America (ISSN 0899-5885) is published quarterly by Elsevier Inc., 360 Park Avenue South, New York, NY 10010-1710. Months of issue are March, June, September, and December. Business and Editorial Offices: 1600 John F. Kennedy Blvd., Suite 1800, Philadelphia, PA 19103-2899. Periodicals postage paid at New York, NY and additional mailing offices. Subscription prices are $144.00 per year for US individuals, $296.00 per year for US institutions, $76.00 per year for US students and residents, $192.00 per year for Canadian individuals, $371.00 per year for Canadian institutions, $219.00 per year for international individuals, $371.00 per year for international institutions and $111.00 per year for Canadian and foreign students/residents. To receive student/resident rate, orders must be accompanied by name of affiliated institution, data of term, and the *signature* of program/ residency coordinator on institution letterhead. Orders will be billed at individual rate until proof of status is received. Foreign air speed delivery is included in all *Clinics* subscription prices. All prices are subject to change without notice. **POSTMASTER:** Send address changes to *Critical Care Nursing Clinics of North America*, Elsevier Health Sciences Division, Subscription Customer Service, 3251 Riverport Lane, Maryland Heights, MO 63043. **Customer Service: 1-800-654-2452 (US and Canada); 314-447-8871 (outside US and Canada). Fax: 314-447-8029. E-mail: JournalsCustomerService-usa@elsevier.com (for print support) and JournalsOnlineSupport-usa@elsevier.com (for online support).**

Reprints. For copies of 100 or more of articles in this publication, please contact the Commercial Reprints Department, Elsevier Inc., 360 Park Avenue South, New York, New York, 10010-1710; Tel.: (212) 633-3813, Fax: (212) 462-1935, and E-mail: reprints@elsevier.com.

Critical Care Nursing Clinics of North America is covered in *MEDLINE/PubMed (Index Medicus), International Nursing Index, Nursing Citation Index, Cumulative Index to Nursing and Allied Health Literature,* and *RNdex Top 100.*

Printed and bound by CPI Group (UK) Ltd, Croydon, CR0 4YY
Transferred to Digital Print 2011

Contributors

CONSULTING EDITOR

JANET FOSTER, PhD, CNS
Texas Woman's University, College of Nursing, Houston, Texas

GUEST EDITOR

BARBARA "BOBBI" LEEPER, MN, RN-BC, CNS M-S, CCRN, FAHA
Clinical Nurse Specialist, Cardiovascular Services, Baylor University Medical Center, Dallas, Texas

AUTHORS

SHEILA BOLANOS, BSN, RN, CCRN
Staff Nurse, The Heart Hospital Baylor Plano, Plano, Texas

MAE M. CENTENO, DNP, RN, CCRN, CCNS, ACNS-BC
Program Manager/Clinical Nurse Specialist, Heart Failure Program and Advanced Lung Disease Center, Baylor University Medical Center, Dallas, Texas

MARIVIC DELA CRUZ, BSN, RN
Staff Nurse, The Heart Hospital Baylor Plano, Plano, Texas

NATALIE CULPEPPER, BSN, RN, CCRN
Staff Nurse, The Heart Hospital Baylor Plano, Plano, Texas

ALAINA M. CYR, BSN, RN, CAPA, NE-BC
Magnet Coordinator, The Heart Hospital Baylor Plano, Plano, Texas; and Clinical Faculty, College of Nursing, The University of Texas at Arlington, Arlington, Texas

ERIKA DINIZ-BORKAR, BSN, RN
Staff Nurse, The Heart Hospital Baylor Plano, Plano, Texas

SONYA FLANDERS, MSN, RN, ACNS-BC, CCRN
Clinical Nurse Specialist, Internal Medicine Services, Baylor University Medical Center, Dallas, Texas

CATHERINE FUSILIER, BSN, RN
Staff Nurse, The Heart Hospital Baylor Plano, Plano, Texas

REBECCA GILLIAM, BSN, RN
Staff Nurse, The Heart Hospital Baylor Plano, Plano, Texas

SHARON GUNN, MSN, MA, RN, ACNS-BC, CCRN
Clinical Nurse Specialist, Critical Care Services, Baylor University Medical Center, Dallas, Texas

CAROL HINKLE, MSN, RN-BC
Education Consultant-Critical Care, Education Department, Brookwood Medical Center, Birmingham, Alabama

PATRICIA A. HUGHES, MSN, RN, CNRN
Stroke Nurse Clinician, Baylor University Medical Center, Dallas, Texas

LEA JOHANNA HYVARINEN, BSN, RN
Staff Nurse, The Heart Hospital Baylor Plano, Plano, Texas

CHRISTA LAMBERT, BSN, RN, CEN
Nurse Manager, Emergency Department and Float Pool; Chest Pain Center Coordinator, The Heart Hospital Baylor Plano, Plano, Texas

PAUL ST. LAURENT, MSN, APRN-BC, ACNP, CCRN
Acute Care Nurse Practitioner, Baylor Hamilton Heart and Vascular Hospital, Dallas, Texas

BARBARA LEEPER, MN, RN-BC, CNS M-S, CCRN, FAHA
Clinical Nurse Specialist, Cardiovascular Services, Baylor University Medical Center, Dallas, Texas

DOUG LONG, BSN, RN, CCRN
Staff Nurse, The Heart Hospital Baylor Plano, Plano, Texas

KIMBERLEE MARTIN, RN
Nurse Supervisor, Emergency Department, The Heart Hospital Baylor Plano, Plano, Texas

SUZANNE MATSON, RN, CCRN
Nurse Manager, The Heart Hospital Baylor Plano, Plano, Texas

MARGARET E. McATEE, MN, RN, ACNP-BC, CCRN
Baylor All Saints Medical Center, Fort Worth, Texas

LAARNI MENDOZA, BSN, RN, CCRN
Staff Nurse, The Heart Hospital Baylor Plano, Plano, Texas

CHARMAINE MOORE, MBA/MHSM, RN
Staff Nurse, The Heart Hospital Baylor Plano, Plano, Texas

CECILIA MORA, BSN, RN, CCRN
Staff Nurse, The Heart Hospital Baylor Plano, Plano, Texas

MALLORY PIASCHYK, MSN, RN
Clinical Nursing Supervisor, The Heart Hospital Baylor Plano, Plano, Texas

TABITHA SOUTH, BSN, RN
Director, Critical Care Services, Baylor Regional Medical Center at Grapevine, Grapevine, Texas

SERENA STANSBURY, BSN, RN
Staff Nurse, The Heart Hospital Baylor Plano, Plano, Texas

ANI TAN, BSN, RN, CCRN
Staff Nurse, The Heart Hospital Baylor Plano, Plano, Texas

AMY WETZEL, BSN, RN
Staff Nurse, The Heart Hospital Baylor Plano, Plano, Texas

Contents

Acute Coronary Syndrome   547

Barbara Leeper, Alaina M. Cyr, Christa Lambert, and Kimberlee Martin

> Cardiovascular disease affects 82.6 million Americans and represents a
> tremendous financial burden for individuals as well as the country.
> Acute coronary syndrome (ACS), one component of cardiovascular
> disease, impacts more than 17 million Americans annually. ACS com-
> prises a spectrum of atherosclerosis including unstable angina, non-
> ST-elevation myocardial infarction (NSTEMI), and ST-segment eleva-
> tion myocardial infarction (STEMI). Early recognition, early treatment,
> decreasing risk factors, and secondary prevention decrease mortality.
> This article describes the spectrum of ACS, management of ACS, and
> secondary prevention strategies.

Acute Coronary Syndrome: New and Evolving Therapies   559

Paul St. Laurent

> Coronary heart disease (CHD) death rates have fallen from 1968 to
> the present, which is attributed to medical and surgical treatments
> as well as changes in the risk factors for cardiovascular disease. It is
> estimated that approximately 25% of this reduction is due to
> advances in the initial treatment and secondary preventive therapies
> after myocardial infarction, as well as revascularization for chronic
> angina. As these therapies continue to evolve, clinicians must stay
> current in their understanding of how this will impact patients and
> alter clinical outcomes.

Coronary Artery Bypass Surgery   573

Tabitha South

> Coronary artery bypass graft (CABG) surgery is a dynamic procedure
> utilized for several decades to alleviate the effects of various processes
> on the coronary arteries. Technological advances coupled with evolving
> surgical expertise continue to mold the CABG procedure and help
> improve quality of life and life expectancy for many patients. As a result,
> ongoing education and research must be done in this field to stay on
> top of the latest innovations. This need to keep up and stay ahead is
> addressed in this article through an increased awareness of surgical
> modalities, treatment options, and patient outcome optimization.

> Valve replacement with cardiopulmonary bypass is currently the treat-
> ment of choice for symptomatic aortic, pulmonic, tricuspid, and mitral
> stenosis and regurgitation but carries a significant risk of morbidity and
> mortality, particularly in patients with comorbidities. Recent medical
> advances have made heart and valve surgeries less complicated,
> greatly reducing morbidity and mortality and allowing shorter recovery
> times. Today these surgeries are performed at younger ages than
> before. Current options for valve replacement and repair allow for the
> most appropriate procedure based on the age and comorbidities of the
> patient. This article discusses heart valve surgery, including nursing
> implications and patient education.

> Treatment for acute myocardial infarction has changed over the past
> few decades. Cardiogenic shock, on the other hand, still carries a high
> risk for mortality. Treatment is based on guidelines and is aimed at
> improving coronary and tissue perfusion to improve cardiac function.
> Interventions include rapid reperfusion therapy as well as pharmaco-
> logic agents and mechanical circulatory support. This article provides a
> review of the current understanding of the etiologies, pathophysiology,
> and recommendations for management of cardiogenic shock.

> Intrinsic and extrinsic risk factors put hospitalized patients at risk for
> pulmonary complications. Potentially serious complications include
> pulmonary embolism and ventilator-induced lung injury. Using a
> case study approach, this report focuses on evidence-based clinical
> strategies for preventing, diagnosing, and treating these problems.
> Important nursing implications aimed at optimizing patient outcomes
> are included.

> Cardiac patients can have a variety of co-morbidities including electro-
> lyte disorders while in the critical care unit. Disorders of potassium,
> magnesium and calcium are the most common. However, disorders of

sodium and phosphorus can also affect cardiac patients. This article discusses electrolyte disorders and their effects upon the cardiovascular system. Electrocardiographic changes related to electrolyte disorders are discussed along with monitoring and treatment.

FORTHCOMING ISSUES

March 2012

Pulmonary, Part I
Kathi Ellstrom, PhD, RN, ACNS-BC,
Guest Editor

June 2012

Pulmonary, Part II
Kathi Ellstrom, PhD, RN, ACNS-BC,
Guest Editor

September 2012

Psychiatric Care
Susan Mace Weeks, DNP, RN, CNS, LMFT,
LCDC, *Guest Editor*

December 2012

Winter Trauma
Margaret Ecklund, MS, RN, CCRN,
ACNP-BC, *Guest Editor*

RECENT ISSUES

September 2011

Transplant
Darlene Lovasik, RN, MN, CCRN, CNRN,
Guest Editor

June 2011

Pediatric Illnesses and Transition of Care
Vicki L. Zeigler, PhD, RN,
Guest Editor

March 2011

Sepsis
R. Phillip Dellinger, MD, MSc,
Guest Editor

THE CLINICS ARE NOW AVAILABLE ONLINE!

Access your subscription at:
www.theclinics.com

Preface

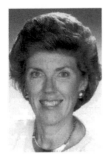

Barbara "Bobbi" Leeper, MN, RN-BC, CNS M-S, CCRN
Guest Editor

This issue of *Critical Care Nursing Clinics* provides a comprehensive review and update of some of the significant cardiovascular disease patient issues we are dealing with today. We know that cardiovascular disease is a major health problem not only for the United States but globally, representing a significant financial burden. The content in this issue addresses clinical practice related to the patient with cardiovascular disease. The issue begins with a review of acute coronary syndromes and a brief review of the atherosclerotic process followed by important aspects for the management of angina, non-ST-segment elevation myocardial infarction, and ST-segment elevation myocardial infarction. The next article brings us forward with new and evolving therapies for acute coronary syndromes. For those patients who require a surgical intervention, there is an overview of coronary artery bypass surgery, which is helpful for those who do not routinely care for these patients. Heart valve surgery is discussed beginning with where we are today and transitioning to invasive transcatheter aortic valve replacement, which is likely to become standard practice as technology evolves.

General topics that are always a challenge when caring for the patient with cardiovascular disease are cardiogenic shock, pulmonary issues focusing on pulmonary embolism and ventilator-induced lung injury, electrolyte disorders, and glucose control. The latest information about caring for a patient with pulmonary hypertension is provided as well as information about comprehensive care of adults with ischemic stroke. Many facilities are seeking certification for stroke. This article provides key information related to that process.

It is hoped that the readers of this issue will find content within that will help them in some aspect of their practice, whether they are pursuing certification, looking for articles to help with orienting new staff to a cardiac ICU, or searching for

Crit Care Nurs Clin N Am 23 (2011) ix–x
doi:10.1016/j.ccell.2011.10.002
0899-5885/11/$ – see front matter © 2011 Elsevier Inc. All rights reserved.

ccnursing.theclinics.com

evidenced-based practices. There's something in this issue for almost every nurse caring for a patient with cardiovascular disease.

Barbara "Bobbi" Leeper, MN, RN-BC, CNS M-S, CCRN
Cardiovascular Services
Baylor University Medical Center
3500 Gaston Avenue
Dallas, TX 75246, USA

E-mail address:
Bobbi.Leeper@baylorhealth.edu

Acute Coronary Syndrome

Barbara Leeper, MN, RN-BC, CNS M-S, CCRN[a],*,
Alaina M. Cyr, BSN, RN, CAPA, NE-BC[b,c], Christa Lambert, BSN, RN, CEN[b],
Kimberlee Martin, RN[b]

KEYWORDS

- Acute coronary syndrome • Coronary
- ST-segment elevation myocardial infarction • Angina
- Heart • Cardiac

At present, cardiovascular disease affects 82.6 million Americans, with more than 8 million Americans experiencing a myocardial infarction (MI) annually. More than 800,000 will succumb to the effects of cardiovascular disease.[1] Although the death rate attributable to cardiovascular disease has declined, it is still the primary cause of death in the United States, accounting for approximately 34% of all deaths.[1] According to the American Heart Association, an American dies from cardiovascular disease every 39 seconds.[1] A recent policy statement from the American Heart Association predicted 40.5% of the population in the United States will have some form of cardiovascular disease, including hypertension, coronary heart disease, heart failure, or stroke.[2] Mortality from cardiovascular disease is estimated to reach 23.4 million by the year 2030. Annually in the United States, an estimated $165.4 billion in direct and indirect costs of cardiovascular disease are realized, with projections of $818 billion in 2030.[2] Hospital emergency departments are inundated on a daily basis with patients presenting with a variety of symptoms. Patients presenting with cardiac symptoms are in need of rapid assessment, diagnosis, and treatment. The following content describes the spectrum of acute coronary syndrome (ACS), management of ACS, and secondary prevention strategies.

OVERVIEW OF ATHEROSCLEROSIS

Acute coronary syndrome (ACS) represents a spectrum of the atherosclerotic process including unstable angina, non-ST-segment elevation MI (NSTEMI), and ST-segment elevation MI (STEMI). It is associated with increased risk of acute myocardial

---

The authors have nothing to disclose.

[a] Cardiovascular Services, Baylor University Medical Center, 3500 Gaston Avenue, Dallas, TX 75246, USA

[b] The Heart Hospital Baylor Plano, 1100 Allied Drive, Plano, TX 75093, USA

[c] College of Nursing, The University of Texas at Arlington, 411 South Nedderman Drive, Arlington, TX 76019, USA

* Corresponding author.

E-mail address: Bobbi.Leeper@baylorhealth.edu

infarction (AMI) and cardiac death.[3] These life-threatening disorders are a major cause of emergency care and hospitalization in the United States.

Although other conditions may lead to the development of angina, the most common cause is atherosclerosis. Atherosclerosis is a disease of the medium and large arteries. The earliest manifestation of atherosclerosis begins in childhood and is characterized by the presence of fatty streaks in the walls of the arteries. The atherosclerotic process begins with injury to the endothelial cells lining the artery. Inflammation ensues, with the accumulation of lipids, cholesterol, calcium, and cellular debris within the intima of the vessel wall. Over time, this process leads to the buildup of these materials protruding into the lumen of the coronary artery, forming an advanced lesion called "fibrous plaque" that usually appears in early adulthood and progresses with age.[4] Unless the plaque ruptures, the patient can remain asymptomatic for a long time. If the plaque ruptures, the platelets become activated and aggregate at the site of the rupture. The intrinsic clotting cascade is activated, resulting in the formation of a thrombus at the site that may cause either fixed occlusion of the vessel or intermittent occlusion. Over time, the thrombus is resorbed and the plaque continues to enlarge. This process may be repeated several times until there is significant obstruction of the coronary artery leading to the onset of symptoms.

The plaque may be described as stable or unstable. The stable plaque does not rupture but continues to increase in size, eventually reducing blood flow and leading to the development of angina. The unstable plaque is also referred to as a vulnerable plaque that is prone to rupture. Triggers for plaque rupture have been found to have a circadian rhythm, occurring more often in the morning. Plaque rupture is also associated with seasonal variation, specifically in the winter, and is often associated with emotional stress or exertion.

SIGNS AND SYMPTOMS

The patient begins experiencing symptoms when the coronary artery becomes so narrowed that blood supply is insufficient to meet the metabolic demands of the cardiac muscle cells, causing ischemia of the myocytes. The symptoms often begin with exertion, which can be in the form of emotional or physical stress. The typical signs and symptoms may include discomfort in the jaw, neck, one or both arms, chest tightness or heaviness, and complaints of shortness of breath. It is important for the clinician to differentiate the signs and symptoms associated with angina from those associated with AMI. Refer to **Box 1** for additional signs and symptoms associated with angina and AMI. A patient experiencing angina will usually have resolution of the discomfort with termination of exertion or after administration of nitroglycerin. The patient experiencing an AMI will have discomfort or pain lasting longer than 20 minutes that usually is not relieved by nitroglycerin. Other signs may include diaphoresis, nausea and vomiting, tachycardia, and shortness of breath. Patients may also report a feeling of impending doom or general feeling of not being well.[3] Women in the throes of experiencing an MI may not have complaints of chest discomfort. Instead, they are likely to have more subtle symptoms such as fatigue and indigestion. The symptom of dyspnea should not be overlooked. Studies have shown self-reported dyspnea in patients undergoing stress perfusion testing was an independent predictor of cardiac and total mortality. The risk of sudden cardiac death was increased fourfold even when patients had no prior history of coronary artery disease.[5]

It is important to keep in mind that not all patients with myocardial ischemia experience chest discomfort.[3] The Framingham Study revealed that in as many as

---

Box 1
Signs and symptoms associated with angina and AMI

Anginal Equivalent:

Resolve with rest OR nitroglycerin

Pain or discomfort

  Jaw

  Neck

  Ear

  Arm

  Epigastric

  Shortness of breath

Acute MI:

Symptoms last longer than 20–30 minutes

Typical

  Tightness

  Chest pain or pressure

  Squeezing

  Heaviness

  Usually lasts longer than 20–30 minutes

  Usually unrelieved by nitroglycerin

May radiate

  Down one or both arms

  Jaw

  Neck

  Back

  Shoulder(s)

Possible associated signs and symptoms

  Dyspnea

  Diaphoresis

  Nausea

  Vomiting

  Light-headedness

  Syncope

---

half of all patients experiencing an MI the symptoms may be clinically silent and unrecognized by the patient.[6] A study looking at patients in the National Registry of Myocardial Infarction (NRMI) found that nearly one-third of patients with confirmed MI had symptoms other than chest pain when presenting to the hospital. When the investigators looked at those MI patients without chest discomfort, the patients were more likely to be older, female, and have diabetes or heart failure or both.[7] The investigators found MI patients without chest pain delayed longer before going to the hospital (mean, 7.9 hours vs 5.3 hours). They were less likely to be diagnosed with an MI on admission (22.2% vs 50.3%) as well as receive evidence-based interventions including thrombolysis or a percutaneous coronary intervention (PCI), aspirin (ASA), beta blockers, or heparin.[7] Patients with "silent" MIs were 2.2 times more likely to die during their hospital stay, with an in-hospital mortality rate of 23.3% when compared to 9.3% for those with a "symptomatic" MI. Clinicians should be cautious to avoid allowing the severity of pain to be a factor in evaluating patients with ACS.[8]

Unstable Angina

Unstable angina is present when there is progression from a stable coronary artery disease state to an unstable disease state. There are three classifications of unstable angina: (1) angina at rest; (2) new onset angina (<2 months); and (3) increasing angina that increases in intensity, duration, or frequency, or all of these.[3] Unstable angina can progress to NSTEMI and STEMI if left untreated. Unstable angina does indicate a reduction in the blood flow in the coronary arteries typically caused by a rupture of atherosclerotic plaque, leading to thrombus formation.[9–11] Studies have shown the average patient experiencing unstable angina delays seeking medical attention as much as 2 hours after symptom onset.[3] A common reason stated by patients for treatment delay is that they expected to have severe crushing chest pain, which is in contrast to what they actually were experiencing.[3]

Unstable angina is diagnosed after STEMI and NSTEMI are ruled out in patients presenting with signs or symptoms of myocardial ischemia. The electrocardiogram (ECG) in patients with unstable angina may demonstrate transient ST-segment depression that develops during the ischemic episode and resolves when the patient's symptoms subside. The cardiac biomarkers will remain within normal limits in patients with unstable angina.

NSTEMI

NSTEMI results when the coronary artery is partially occluded causing myocardial cell death. This type of MI occurs more frequently than STEMI. These patients will demonstrate a minor elevation of their cardiac biomarker. Their ECG will demonstrate abnormal ST-segment depression or prominent T-wave inversion or both.[3,10,12] **Fig. 1** is an example of a NSTEMI. Patients with a NSTEMI will not go on to develop ST-segment elevation on their ECG.

STEMI

STEMI occurs when there is an abrupt and complete occlusion of the coronary artery causing acute ischemia. STEMI is the most serious form of ACS with the highest rate of mortality.[13] The classic finding on the ECG is ST-segment elevation (**Fig. 2**). The cardiac biomarkers are elevated above normal, and in some cases can be linked to the timing of the acute closure of the vessel.

MANAGEMENT OF ACS

Patients arriving at the emergency department triage desk should be rapidly assessed for signs and symptoms of ACS and immediately taken to a room. A 12-lead ECG should be obtained quickly and interpreted in a timely manner. This is vital to identification of patients in need of reperfusion treatment.[14] Guidelines recommend obtaining an initial ECG within 10 minutes of presentation and continuous ECG monitoring for patients with suspected STEMI.[13]

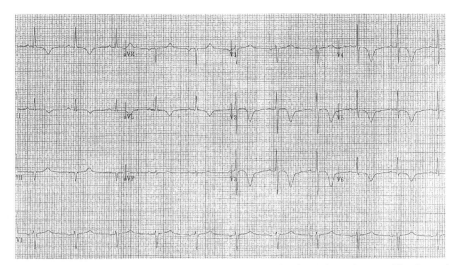

Fig. 1. NSTEMI. Note the prominent T-wave inversion in leads V2 through V5 and leads I and avL indicative of an anterior lateral infarction. This ECG was recorded on a 68-year-old woman within 6 minutes of arriving at the emergency department.

Cardiac biomarkers should be drawn and sent to the laboratory as soon as possible. The biomarkers are useful for diagnosing/correlating with time of symptom onset. When the cardiac myocytes are ischemic for a sustained period of time, the cell membranes lose their integrity and macromolecules will diffuse out into the circulation and eventually become detectable. The common biomarkers used in clinical practice include the serum troponin I and T, and creatine kinase MB (CK-MB). The CK-MB is the first to rise, usually within 3 to 6 hours of symptom onset. It is followed by troponin

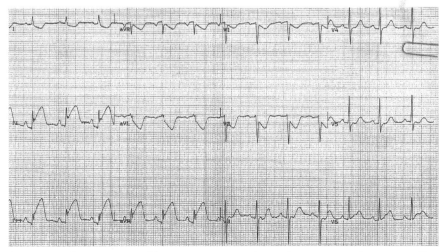

Fig. 2. STEMI from a 54-year-old man upon presentation to the emergency department. Note the elevated ST-segments in leads II, III, and avF.

I and T. Evaluation of serum troponin I is very cardiac specific and one of the best indicators for myocardial injury. Troponin I begins to rise within 3 to 6 hours after symptom onset and peaks at 12 hours.[15] One of the advantages of troponin I for diagnosis of AMI is that it will remain elevated for as long at 5 to 10 days after the MI. This is useful for diagnosing an MI in patients who may delay coming to the hospital for as long as 3 to 4 days.

MANAGEMENT OF PATIENTS WITH ACS

Management of ACS begins at the initial point of contact with a health care provider and should be based on predetermined written protocols.[13] The management of ACS includes pain relief, early reperfusion, use of antiplatelet therapy and anticoagulants, controlling the risk factors, and secondary prevention. There are similarities in the management of patients with ACS, but there are also differences. Each is discussed in the following section.

Unstable Angina/NSTEMI

The management of patients experiencing unstable angina/NSTEMI should have two immediate goals including the immediate relief of chest discomfort and prevention of serious adverse outcomes. The achievement of these goals includes the initiation of anti-ischemic therapy, antithrombotic therapy, and invasive procedures. Patients with ongoing symptoms should be admitted to a coronary care unit for closer monitoring and ready access to PCI.[3] Those who are asymptomatic after interventions have been found to do well on cardiac telemetry units with continuous ECG monitoring.

The standards indicate the administration of oxygen as well as restricted activity levels will increase oxygen delivery to the myocardium and reduce cardiac workload. Morphine is administered intravenously and titrated according to response to provide pain relief. The typical dosage is 2 to 4 mg intravenously (IV) with increments of 2 to 8 mg IV repeated at 5- to 15-minute intervals. Morphine works directly on the nervous system to reduce anxiety and lessen the autonomic responses such as diaphoresis associated with MI. In addition, morphine has a slight effect on dilation of the coronary arteries to increase oxygen supply to the cardiac tissue.[16]

Anti-ischemic therapy includes the administration of nitroglycerin IV, sublingually, or by nasal spray. Nitroglycerin dilates the venous bed and increases venous pooling, thus reducing venous return (preload) to the heart. This contributes to a further reduction of myocardial work, restoring the balance between oxygen delivery and oxygen demand. Nitro spray is short acting with effects lasting up to 30 minutes. The sublingual route is preferred owing to the avoidance of metabolism in the liver.[16] Nitrates should not be administered if the systolic blood pressure is less than 90 mm Hg or to patients who have received a phosphodiesterase inhibitor for erectile dysfunction in the last 24 to 48 hours.[13]

Antiplatelet medications work to prevent thrombus formation and reduce the risk of subsequent MI, stroke, and death. Currently, aspirin and clopidogrel are the most often used antiplatelet medications.[17] Aspirin is recommended for all patients presenting with signs and symptoms of ACS. Patients should be given 325 mg of aspirin orally upon presentation of chest discomfort if there are no contraindications. Having a patient chew the aspirin allows for a more rapid buccal absorption. Aspirin inhibits the formation of thrombus by inhibiting thromboxane A_2 production. The administration of aspirin as a first-line treatment decreases the rate of cardiovascular death by up to one half. The ongoing usage of aspirin is recommended for patients who have suffered a cardiac event if there are no contraindications.[13,17]

The use of clopidogrel, in addition to aspirin, is part of the standard regimen for NSTEMI patients. Clopidogrel works to block adenosine diphosphate receptor sites, preventing platelet aggregation. Adenosine diphosphate is produced by platelets and attaches to receptor sites on the surface of platelets to promote platelet aggregation.[18]

Another class of platelet inhibitors is the glycoprotein IIbIIIa inhibitors. These primarily include abciximab (Reopro) and eptifibatide (Integrilin). These medications may be initiated before a PCI, and in some cases are continued for several hours after the interventional procedure.[16] Their primary effect is to inhibit platelet aggregation and prevent abrupt vessels closure, especially after a stent has been deployed.

Anticoagulation is a first-line therapy for NSTEMI and unstable angina. Anticoagulation therapy is utilized in STEMI in conjunction with other interventions. Anticoagulants include heparin and enoxaparin, a low molecular weight heparin. Heparin reduces thrombus formation by blocking thrombin production. Low molecular weight heparin such as enoxaparin is administered subcutaneously and does not require laboratory monitoring.[19,20] Bleeding is a potential complication of anticoagulation therapy. Reducing the risk for bleeding is accomplished through weight-adjusted dosing, modified dosing in patients with renal dysfunction, or selection of an alternate therapy in patient at higher risk for bleeding.[20]

Early beta blockade has been shown to reduce mortality and recurrent MIs. Beta blockers decrease myocardial oxygen consumption. Short-acting beta blockers such as metoprolol are used initially if there are no contradictions. Long-acting beta blockers decrease the heart rate and contribute to reducing oxygen demands of the cardiac muscle. Beta blockers are the only class of drugs that have been shown to reduce the incidence of sudden cardiac death after MI. It is important that the beta blocker be initiated while the patient is hospitalized rather than wait to start it during a follow-up visit with the health care provider. A delay in initiation (after discharge) has been shown to be less effective in reducing sudden cardiac death. Calcium channel blockers are used in patients who may not tolerate or have contraindications to beta blockers.[15]

Angiotensin-converting enzyme (ACE) inhibitors should be initiated within the first 24 hours after an MI, particularly if the left ventricular ejection fraction is less than 40%. ACE inhibitors prevent the conversion of angiotensin I to angiotensin II. Angiotensin II causes peripheral vasoconstriction and is thought to contribute to the development of hypertrophy of the myocytes adjacent to the infarcted tissue, which may contribute to the development of a ventricular aneurysm after MI. Side effects of ACE inhibitors include hypotension, cough, and angioedema. Angioedema refers to swelling of the lower portion of the face externally or can involve the oropharynx, compromising the patient's airway. Patients should be monitored for this potentially life-threatening side effect regularly. ACE inhibitors may prevent the development of ventricular hypertrophy and ventricular aneurysm.[16]

STEMI

The American Heart Association/American College of Cardiology (AHA/ACC) standards for the management of acute STEMI recommend immediate reperfusion once the diagnosis of STEMI is made. Reperfusion strategies include the use of fibrinolytics or primary coronary intervention. Nielsen and colleagues examined the effects of system delay and timing of interventions for AMI.[21] They found system delays contribute to incremental increases in 30-day and 8-year mortality for both fibrinolysis and primary PCI. If primary PCI was achieved within 2 hours, mortality rates were lower when compared to early fibrinolysis. System delays for primary PCI greater than

3 hours was associated with similar mortality when fibrinolysis was administered within 1 to 2 hours. The investigators concluded primary PCI is preferred to early fibrinolysis up to 2 hours after the first contact with a health care provider. One also must consider individual patient characteristics.[21]

The AHA/ACC standards clearly state that patients presenting with STEMI to a facility without the capability for timely intervention with PCI within 90 minutes should undergo fibrinolysis.[13] The fibrinolytic should be administered within 30 minutes of arrival to the emergency department. The common agents used currently include retaplase and tenectplase. Both can be administered IV in single doses. Their ease of administration has replaced the administration of a 90-minute infusion of atelplase for the acute management of STEMI.

Early reperfusion through PCI reduces mortality by 25% and is the treatment of choice, as indicated previously.[18,19] Mechanical reperfusion using primary PCI should occur within 90 minutes of presentation to the hospital (door-to-balloon time).[13] This usually occurs in the form of balloon angioplasty. A stent may be inserted to maintain the patency of the vessel. Successful reperfusion has occurred when there is at least a 50% reduction in ST-elevation.[13] A recent report demonstrated a decline in door-to-balloon time from a median of 96 minutes to 64 minutes from 2005 to 2010.[22] Patients who do not achieve successful reperfusion with PCI may need a coronary artery bypass grafting (CABG).

IMPLICATIONS FOR NURSING

STEMI patients should be admitted to a unit that has continuous ECG and pulse oximetry monitoring and the ability for hemodynamic monitoring such as a coronary care unit or intensive care unit after the reperfusion intervention.[13,14] Low-risk STEMI patients and other types of ACS patients may be admitted to step-down or telemetry units.[9] All patients with ACS should have continuous ECG monitoring.[23]

The aim of continuous ECG monitoring is to observe for dysrhythmias as well as ECG signs of acute closure involving the target vessel(s). This may be manifested by ST-segment changes on the cardiac monitor. The current practice standards recommend monitoring in the lead(s) that have been found to be most sensitive for recording ischemic changes in a particular area of the heart.[23] For example, if the lesion was in the right coronary artery affecting the left ventricular inferior wall, lead III is the most sensitive lead for ischemic changes. If the left anterior descending coronary artery was involved, lead V3 is the best lead for monitoring. Lead V5 has been found to be the best lead for monitoring for ischemic changes associated with the lateral wall and circumflex coronary artery.[23]

The level of activity of hospitalized ACS patients begins with bedrest and commode or bathroom privileges for the first 24 hours after admission. Once the patient is free of recurrent discomfort, symptoms of heart failure, or serious heart rhythm disturbances, the patient can begin to increase activity levels and is eligible to begin a cardiac rehabilitation regimen.[13] Today, the average length of stay for an AMI patient is approximately 3 days. This short length of stay often presents a challenge for the nurse to provide effective patient/family education.

Secondary Prevention: Controlling Risk Factors

Prevention of reoccurring cardiac events can be addressed through risk factor modification. Once a patient has a cardiac event, the factors to reduce that reoccurrence are called secondary prevention factors. Reducing a patient's risk for further cardiac events is vital. Strategies include medical and lifestyle management. Medical management includes the following medications on discharge: beta blocker,

---

Box 2
Indicators for AMI core measure

1. First EKG within 10 minutes of arrival

2. Aspirin on arrival and prescribed discharge

3. Fibrinolytic administered within 30 minutes of arrival if applicable

4. Primary PCI performed within 90 minutes of arrival if applicable

5. Adult smoking cessation/advice/counseling

6. Beta blocker prescribed at discharge

7. ACE inhibitor at discharge if left ventricular ejection fraction < 40%

8. Statin prescribed at discharge

ACE inhibitor if the left ventricular EF is less than 40%, lipid lowering agent as appropriate, and aspirin. Clopidogrel will be prescribed if the patient has had a stent deployed during the PCI procedure. Patients must be taught the importance of continuing to take both the aspirin and clopidogrel as prescribed by the physician. Failure to continue with the clopidogrel can lead to abrupt closure of the stent and subsequent MI. Patients should always contact their health care provider if they have any question about their medications.

Patients should be screened and monitored for the presence and status of risk factors.[13] Tobacco cessation, control of hypertension, and management of diabetes have been shown to have the biggest impact on reducing cardiovascular disease. Lifestyle risk factors that should also be addressed in addition to those mentioned previously, include lowering total cholesterol to less than 200 mg/dL, increasing high density lipoprotein (HDL) levels to greater than 50 to 60 mg/dL, and lowering low-density lipoprotein (LDL) cholesterol to less than 120 mg/dL.[3]

Cardiac rehabilitation assists patients to adjust to lifestyle changes and provides guidelines for an exercise and activity regimen. Patients should gradually increase physical exercise to 30 to 45 minutes per day for at least 5 days a week. Nutritional counseling can provide a framework for appropriate choices including foods low in saturated fats, sodium, *trans*-fatty acids, and cholesterol. Weight management is important for long-term cardiovascular health. The recommended body mass index (BMI) is 18.5 to 24.9 kg/m^2. Weight, diet, and exercise all have an impact on lipid management, blood pressure control, and the demand placed on the heart. Tobacco cessation should be addressed. There are a variety of methods available to reduce the use of tobacco. Management of diabetes decreases the risk for cardiovascular events and death. Patients with diabetes should maintain an HbA$_{1c}$ of less than 7 through diet, lifestyle modification, and medications.[3,9]

Patient education should begin from the first contact with the patient/family through discharge. Before discharge, a referral to cardiac rehabilitation or community support groups is recommended.[3,13] Education should include family members and provide a comprehensive overview of strategies to reduce risk factors. Additional information for the patient and family members should include recognition of cardiac symptoms and appropriate actions to take in case another cardiac event occurs. It is advisable to recommend that family members learn about automatic external defibrillators (AEDs) and cardiopulmonary resuscitation (CPR).[3,13]

SUMMARY

Implementation of the AHA/ACC standards for AMI is crucial for patient management and outcomes. The Centers for Medicare/Medicaid (CMS) has established indicators within the AMI core measure to ensure the evidence-based care is provided during the hospital stay. This core measure includes specific indicators that must be documented in the medical record. Refer to **Box 2** for a list of the indicators.

A recent announcement by the United States Department of Health and Human Services (HHS) stated the United States is declaring war on heart disease.[24] Current costs for treating heart disease and stroke is estimated to be $1 out of every $6 in health care expenditures. This initiative is called the "Million Hearts Initiative." Ten states will receive $85 million in grants for the purpose of addressing chronic diseases targeting weight reduction, smoking cessation, control of lipids, and prevention of diabetes.[24]

Early recognition and early intervention for patients with ACS, followed by management of risk factors with secondary prevention strategies, are key to decreasing ACS-related mortality. Management of the ACS patient does not end with discharge from the hospital, but is continued throughout the patient's lifetime.

REFERENCES

1. Roger V, Go A, Llogy-Jones D, et al. Heart disease and stroke statistics 2011 update: a report from the American Heart Association. Circulation 2011;123:e18–209.
2. Heidenreich PA, Trogdon JG, Khavjou OA, et al. Forecasting the future of cardiovascular disease in the United States: a policy statement from the American Heart Association. Circulation 2011;123(8):933–44.
3. Anderson J, Adams C, Antman E, et al. ACC/AHA 2007 guidelines for the management of patients with unstable angina/non-ST-elevation myocardial infarction: executive summary. Circulation 2007;116:803–77.
4. Moser D, Riegel B. Cardiac nursing: a companion to Braunwald's heart disease. St. Louis (MO): Saunders Elsevier; 2008.
5. Abidov A, Rozanski A, Hachamovitch R, et al. Prognostic significance of dyspnea in patients referred for cardiac stress testing. N Engl J Med 2005;353:1889–98.
6. Kannel WB. Silent myocardial ischemia and infarction: insights from the Framingham Study. Cardiol Clin 1986;4:583–91.
7. Canto JG, Shlipak MG, Rogers WJ, et al. Prevalence, clinical characteristics, and mortality among patients with myocardial infarction presenting without chest pain. JAMA 2000;283:3223–9.
8. Edwards M, Chang AM, Matsura AC, et al. Relationship between pain severity and outcome in patients presenting with potential acute coronary syndromes. Ann Emerg Med 2011. [Epub ahead of print].
9. Cassar A, Holmes DR, Rihal C, et al. Chronic coronary artery disease: diagnosis and management. Mayo Clin Proc 2009;84:1130–46.
10. DeVon HA, Ryan CJ. Chest pain and associated symptoms of acute coronary syndromes. J Cardiovasc Nurs 2005;4:232–8.
11. Overbaugh KJ. Acute coronary syndrome. Am J Nurs 2009;109:42–52.
12. Grenne B, Eek C, Sjoli B, et al. Changes of myocardial function in patients with non-ST-elevation acute coronary syndrome awaiting coronary angiography. Am J Cardiol 2010;105:1212–8.
13. Antman E, Anbe D, Armstrong P, et al. ACC/AHA guidelines for the management of patients with ST-elevation myocardial infarction: executive summary. Circulation 2004;110:588–636.

14. Pelter M, Carey M, Stephens K, et al. Improving nurses' ability to identify anatomic location and leads on 12-lead electrocardiograms with ST elevation myocardial infarction. Eur J Cardiovasc Nurs 2010;9:218–25.
15. Woods SL, Sivarajan Froelicher ES, Motzer SA, et al. Cardiac nursing. 6th edition. Philadelphia: Lippincott, Williams & Wilkins; 2010.
16. Opie LH, Gersh BJ. Drugs for the heart. 7th edition. Philadelphia: Saunders.
17. Spinler SA. Oral antiplatelet therapy after acute coronary syndrome and percutaneous coronary intervention: balancing efficacy and bleeding risk. Am J Health Syst Pharm 2010;67:S7–17.
18. Giugliano RP, Braunwald E. The year in non-ST-segment elevation acute coronary syndrome. JACC 2007;50:1386–95.
19. McFeely JE. Acute coronary syndrome: a concise summary for the non-cardiologist. Crit Care Alert 2009;17(2):14–6.
20. Giugliano RP, Braunwald E. The year in non-ST-segment elevation acute coronary syndrome. JACC 2008;52(3):1095–1108.
21. Nielsen, PH, Terkelsen CJ, Nielsen TT, et al. System delay and timing of intervention in acute myocardial infarction from the Danish Acute Myocardial Infarction-2 [DANAMI-2 Trial]. Am J Cardiol 2011;108(6):776–8.
22. Krumholz HM, Miller HJ, Drye EE, et al. Improvements in door to balloon time in the United States, 2005–2010. Circulation 2011;124(9):1038–45.
23. Drew BJ, Califf RM, Funk M, et al. Practice standards for electrocardiographic monitoring in hospital settings. Circulation 2004;110:2721–46.
24. Thomson R. United States Declares War on Heart Disease. Available at http://reuters.com/assets. Accessed September 14, 2011.

Acute Coronary Syndrome: New and Evolving Therapies

Paul St. Laurent, MSN, APRN-BC, ACNP, CCRN

KEYWORDS

- Coronary artery disease
- Percutaneous coronary intervention • Stent thrombosis
- Transradial access • Antiplatelet therapy • Dyslipidemia

Coronary heart disease (CHD) death rates have fallen from 1968 to the present, which is attributed to medical and surgical treatments as well as changes in the risk factors for cardiovascular disease. It is estimated that approximately 25% of this reduction is due to advances in the initial treatment and secondary preventive therapies after myocardial infarction (MI), as well as revascularization for chronic angina.[1] Risk factor modification, especially the reduction of total cholesterol and blood pressure, and a lower smoking rate, have also made a significant positive impact. This article will explore new and evolving therapies aimed at reducing the mortality and morbidity associated with CHD.

Although the death rate has fallen, CHD continues to be the largest major killer of Americans, causing 1 of every 6 deaths in the United States.[1] Every 25 seconds, an American experiences a coronary event, and every minute, someone dies as a result. This year (2011), almost 1 million Americans will experience an acute MI resulting from CHD. For the majority of these individuals, this will be their first and only event. Approximately one-third of these people, however, will have a recurrent infarction.

In recent years, there has been an explosion of technology and innovation in the treatment of CHD. New tools, techniques, and therapies are needed to treat patients. This article will explore some of the recent advances in the treatment of CHD, as well as look ahead to future therapies that are expected to significantly impact both the mortality and morbidity associated with this pervasive disease.

IN THE BEGINNING

The first successful percutaneous transluminal coronary angioplasty (PTCA) performed on an awake patient occurred in September 1977 in Zurich. Andreas Gruentzig, a German physician working at University Hospital in Switzerland,

The author has nothing to disclose.
Baylor Heart and Vascular Hospital, 621 North Hall Street, Dallas, TX 75226, USA
E-mail address: paulstl@baylorhealth.edu

performed the procedure.[2] The first PTCA performed in the United States occurred the following year in both San Francisco and New York. Initial success rates were poor and complications frequent. Of the first 50 patients who underwent PTCA, the primary success rate was only 64% and emergency coronary artery bypass grafting (CABG) was required in 14%, with a periprocedural MI rate of 6%. With experience, success rates increased to approximately 90%. Within the next few years, the number of PTCA procedures performed in the United States grew exponentially, and by the mid-1980s more than 300,000 procedures were performed annually. According to the most current statistics, 1.2 million percutaneous coronary procedures were performed in the United States in 2007.[1]

Two factors that have limited the long-term success of PTCA are acute vessel closure and restenosis. The underlying causes of these phenomena are secondary to complex processes resulting from balloon inflation and plaque compression.[3] Endothelial denudation with rapid accumulation of platelets and fibrin result from the stretching, fracturing, and fissuring of plaque during balloon inflation.[4] Termed a "controlled injury" by Gruentzig, this triggers an inflammatory response with the proliferation of smooth muscle cells within the vessel called neointima. Neointimal proliferation, or hyperplasia, is one mechanism that is associated with restenosis. Restenosis, defined as more than 50% reduction in postprocedural luminal diameter, often occurs within 6 months after angioplasty.[4] Additional mechanisms associated with the restenotic process include early elastic recoil and negative vessel remodeling.[5] Negative remodeling, or vessel shrinkage, has been shown to contribute to late luminal narrowing after PTCA.[6] Although it has been 30 years since the first angioplasty was performed, rates of restenosis remain at 30%. Another problem associated with angioplasty is acute vessel closure. This can occur within seconds after balloon deflation and is often associated with intimal dissection, acute thrombus formation, or both.[3] The incidence of acute vessel closure is 4% to 9% and is associated with a 10-fold increase in mortality. These unacceptable rates of restenosis lead to the search for a more effective long-term solution.

STENTING

The reported first use of coronary stents in humans was in 1987.[7] The development of the stent addressed 2 of the 3 mechanisms thought to be responsible for restenosis. Both recoil and remodeling were virtually eliminated by the mechanical scaffolding provided by the stent.[5] In 1993, both the Belgium Netherlands Stent Arterial Revascularization Therapies Study (BENESTENT) and North American Stent Restenosis Study (STRESS) confirmed stenting significantly improved angiographic and clinical outcomes and established elective coronary stent implantation as standard of care.[8,9] Bare metal stents (BMS) were approved in the United States in 1993, and by 1999, 84% of all interventions involved stent insertion. As stent placement became the standard of care, the problem of neointimal hyperplasia remained unresolved. In addition, a new problem emerged: stent thrombosis.

STENT THROMBOSIS

Stent thrombosis is the most devastating complication of stent placement and in the majority of patients, results in an ST-elevation myocardial infarction. MI associated with acute stent thrombosis carries 20% mortality.[4] Several factors have been identified that predict the occurrence of stent thrombosis. These include acute coronary syndrome (ACS), left ventricular ejection fraction ≤ 30%, bifurcation treatment, renal insufficiency, diabetes, and premature or standard discontinuation of antiplatelet therapy.[4] Of these, premature discontinuation of antiplatelet therapy remains the strongest independent predictor of stent thrombosis.[4]

Although both BENESTENT and STRESS showed a significant decrease in thrombosis compared with angioplasty, the incidence of MI and death was higher than with balloon angioplasty alone. This was despite a complex anticoagulation regimen consisting of dextran, aspirin, dipyridamole, heparin, and warfarin. A dramatic reduction in stent thrombosis occurred with the use of intravascular ultrasound and high balloon pressures to optimize stent placement. In addition, replacing anticoagulation with dual antiplatelet therapy (DAPT) had a significant and long-term effect on the incidence of stent thrombosis.

DRUG-ELUTING STENTS

It was well understood that neointimal hyperplasia was the primary underlying cause of stent restenosis. This led to the development of the drug-eluting stent (DES). A DES is coated with a polymer-containing antiproliferative material that inhibits neointimal hyperplasia. It was hoped that by inhibiting neointimal hyperplasia, the DES would eliminate restenosis and the need for reintervention. The first-generation DES released sirolimus or paclitaxel from a nonresorbable polymer. These agents inhibited vascular smooth cell migration and proliferation, thereby preventing restenosis. The DES was approved for use in Europe 2002, and in the United States in 2003. This approval was based on studies that showed a reduction in neointimal hyperplasia, restenosis, and reintervention at 6 to 12 months when compared with a BMS. Unfortunately, the reduction in restenosis was overshadowed by the rate of stent thrombosis, which resulted in MIs and death. As researchers began to investigate the underlying causes of stent thrombosis, the evidence demonstrated that incomplete endothelial coverage of the stent struts played a significant role.[10]

ENDOTHELIALIZATION

Endothelialization is a process whereby the exposed metal struts of a newly deployed stent are covered by a layer of endothelial cells. During this process, the stent struts are a potent source for the formation of platelet-rich microthrombi. These microthrombi can proliferate, leading to an occlusive thrombus.[11] A BMS is completely endothelialized in 28 days. A DES, however, takes significantly longer secondary to the antiproliferative properties of the agents used. In a study by Kotani and colleagues, both sirolimus-eluting and BMS were compared at 3 to 6 months after implantation. All BMS were completely endothelialized, whereas 87% of the sirolimus-eluting stents were not. Of these, 50% contained thrombi.[10] In addition, angioscopic findings revealed incomplete healing, fibrin deposition, and inflammatory cells, indicating a hypersensitivity reaction. Although the DES greatly reduced the rate of restenosis, the delayed rate of endothelialization and subsequent risk of late stent thrombosis continued to be of concern.

The development of the DES has been credited with a 50% to 70% decrease in restenosis compared with the BMS.[12] The current generation of the DES incorporates a permanent polymer to delay the release of active compound from the stent platform and enhance anti-restenotic efficacy.[13] The long-term safety of polymer-based DES has been called into question because of concerns about late and very late stent thrombosis secondary to impaired arterial healing, characterized by delayed re-endothelialization and persistence of fibrin. Emerging evidence suggests that polymer residue may promote on ongoing inflammatory response in the vessel wall. This chronic vascular hypersensitivity may lead to late thrombosis, stent occlusion, and neointimal overgrowth.[13,14]

DRUG-ELUTING STENTS: THE NEXT GENERATION

The development of polymer-free stents has become a primary area for new research and development.[15] Given the persistent arterial wall inflammation and delayed vascular healing associated with polymer, it has been hypothesized that a polymer-free stent could significantly impact the incidence of stent thrombosis. Several new technologies have come to the forefront to address this issue. They include the bioabsorbable polymer DES, the polymer-free DES, and the biodegradable stent (BDS).

A bioabsorbable polymer DES consists of a BMS, a drug, and a polymer that biodegrades once it has eluted the drug. Only a BMS is left in place in the vessel. This is one of the most widely developed next-generation stenting technologies. The benefit of this technology is that the polymer ensures controlled drug elution, but then biodegrades after it has served its purpose. There is no polymer or polymer residue left behind, and therefore the risk of stent thrombosis is reduced. It is hypothesized that once the polymer has dissolved, the incidence of polymer-induced inflammation and subsequent thrombosis is reduced. This could eliminate the need for long-term dual antiplatelet drugs, and reduce the attendant risks associated with this therapy. This new technology, however, is not without a down side. Evidence has demonstrated that as the polymer degrades, a significant inflammatory reaction may occur. In addition, the breakdown products may also act as potent mediators of inflammation.[14] Despite these concerns, numerous biodegradable polymer stents are in development. These include the BioMatrix (Biosensors, Morges, Switzerland), Nobori (Terumo, Leuven, Belgium), Supralimus (Sahajanand Medical Technologies, Gujrat, India), JACTAX (Boston Scientific, Natick, MA, USA), NEVO (Cordis, Bridgewater, NJ, USA), and EXCEL (JW Medical Systems, Weihai, China). Among the most interesting of these new stents designs is the NEVO. This stent is an open-cell, cobalt chromium stent, with a biodegradable polymer that elutes sirolimus. Both the polymer and sirolimus are contained within reservoirs, which eliminate the need for a surface polymer coating. This reduces tissue-polymer contact by over 75%.[14] Another stent of note is the EXCEL, coated with sirolimus and a poly-L-lactic acid (PLLA) biodegradable polymer. This polymer completely degrades into carbon dioxide and water in 6 to 9 months, leaving a BMS behind. Recent data from the CREATE (Multi-Center Registry Trial of EXCEL Biodegradable Polymer Drug-Eluting Stent) registry in over 2000 patients showed a stent thrombosis rate of 0.87%, despite 81% of patients discontinuing clopidogrel (Plavix) at 6 months.[15]

Another promising area of development is the polymer-free stent. These stents completely eliminate the use of polymer, which is believed to lead to increased rates of thrombosis.[14] These designs include coatings or surface modification technologies that control drug elution. As with the bioabsorbable polymer stents, polymer-free stents offer the possibility of a shorter length of dual antiplatelet therapy. At present, only 4 companies are developing such a product because of the challenge of maintaining the appropriate rate of drug release in the absence of a polymer to control drug elution. Among the most unique offerings is the YUKON (Translumina, Hechingen, Germany). Made of polymer-free stainless steel, this stent has a microporous surface that functions as a reservoir for rapamycin. The device is coated in a stent-coating machine in the cardiac catheterization laboratory, just before percutaneous coronary intervention (PCI). Three other polymer-free stents currently in clinical trials include the Amazonia Pax (Minvasys, Genevilliers, France), BioFREEDOM (Biosensors International, Singapore), and VESTAsync (MIV, Therapeutics, Vancouver, BC, Canada). Current clinical studies of polymer-free stents are limited, and currently only the YUKON is available commercially in Europe, whereas several others are undergoing initial trials.[14]

BIODEGRADABLE STENTS

The next evolution in stent design is the BDS, which is completely dissolvable. The BDS provides the initial scaffolding needed by the vessel to reduce restenosis, but then dissolves, leaving a natural, healed vessel. With nothing left behind, there are no triggers for thrombosis such as a non-endothelialized stent strut, or drug polymer. Similar to a bioabsorbable polymer and polymer-free stent, the BDS may also reduce the need for long-term antiplatelet therapy. The main challenge is to develop a suitable material that provides the initial strength required, but does not dissolve too quickly or fail on deployment.[14]

Current BDS are composed of a polymer or metal alloy. Numerous polymers are available, each with a different chemical composition and bioabsorption time. PLLA, which is also used in many of the biodegradable polymer stents, is metabolized via the Krebs cycle into carbon dioxide (CO_2) and water (H_2O) in a 12- to 18-month period. PLLA is already used clinically in resorbable sutures and soft tissue and orthopedic implants. The AMS-1 BDS (Biotronik, Berlin, Germany) is a biodegradable metallic stent made from magnesium. It degrades in 2 to 3 months, forming inorganic salts containing calcium, chloride, oxide, sulfates, and phosphates.

With the rapid development of new stent technology, a significant question remains unanswered. It is not known whether this new technology will translate into improved clinical outcomes.[16,17] Because only small studies with short-term follow-up have been conducted, the clinical advantages are still unknown. Although the initial results have been promising, more definitive research is needed. For these reasons, large-scale trials with long-term follow-up will be required to determine the clinical efficacy and safety of biodegradable polymer, polymer-free, and biodegradable stents. Another important question is how this new stent technology will impact the need for long-term dual antiplatelet therapy. This is an important clinical issue that will have a significant impact on the management of patients undergoing PCI.

TRANSRADIAL ACCESS

Over 1 million cardiac catheterizations were performed in the United States in 2007, and an estimated 622,000 patients underwent PCI.[1] Although the traditional method of vascular access has been via the femoral artery, this approach is associated with a number of significant vascular complications including access site hematomas, arterial dissections, retroperitoneal bleeds, and pseudoaneurysms. Bleeding complications that occur in the peri-PCI period are associated with worse clinical outcomes and increased mortality rates.[14] Most bleeding events associated with PCI are hematomas at the site of vascular access. Data from the National Heart, Lung, and Blood Institute Dynamic Registry, which included 6656 patients, showed that of all the patients who developed hematomas, 97% underwent transfemoral access.[18] Methods that reduce access site bleeding can have a significant impact on complications and the associated morbidity and mortality that may result.

The percutaneous transradial artery approach for diagnostic coronary angiography was first described by Campeau in 1989.[19] Kiemeneij adapted existing equipment and advanced the use of the radial artery for PCI in the early 1990s. Today, the transradial approach accounts for less than 10% of procedures worldwide, and 1% to 3% of cases in the United States.[20] Although there are several advantages associated with the radial approach, this has been slow to catch on. This is likely because of physicians' familiarity with the femoral or brachial approach, a lack of compatible equipment, as well as the development of femoral closure devices, which have resulted in quicker hemostasis and earlier ambulation.[21,22]

Why Radial?

When considering a change in clinical practice, it is important to weigh the pros and cons of using a new technique, medication, or protocol. A systematic and critical review of the available literature is also crucial to ensure that there is sufficient evidence to support the change. There are several advantages associated with using the transradial approach for coronary angiography. The primary advantage, however, is a significant reduction in vascular complications. A meta-analysis done by Jolly, consisting of 23 randomized trials and more than 7000 patients, demonstrated a reduction in major bleeding by 73% in patients who had radial access compared with those with a femoral approach.[23] Another important advantage of radial access is that the hand has a dual blood supply via the radial and ulnar artery, which limits the potential for limb-threatening ischemia. This technique is advantageous for patients with severe occlusive aortoiliac disease, who otherwise would be amenable to femoral artery cannulation. It is also beneficial for patients with difficulty lying flat because it is not necessary to keep the leg extended, and therefore the head of the bed can be raised without compromising the access site. Increased patient comfort and early ambulation increase patient satisfaction. Early ambulation and reduced complications translate into reduced costs, considering the average cost of a PCI hospitalization without complications is $14,000, and with complications is approximately $27,000.[24]

Patient selection is important to ensure a positive outcome when using the transradial approach. The evaluation process should consist of a thorough history and physical to rule out upper extremity peripheral vascular disease, including Buerger's or Raynaud's disease. In addition, an Allen's test, oximetry, and/or plethysmography should be performed to determine if adequate ulnar arterial perfusion is present. Any abnormalities are contraindications to transradial access. Other things to consider when deciding whether to consider transradial access is whether the patient might require an intra-aortic balloon pump or need the radial artery as a conduit for coronary artery bypass surgery or for future dialysis access. In these scenarios, femoral access is preferred.[25]

A significant operator learning curve exists because of the need to learn a new technique. This learning curve may initially result in higher failure rates, increased radiation exposure, and longer procedures.[25] However, like any new technique, this learning curve can be shortened by a properly implemented training program and optimal access technique.[26] Success rates for experienced operators in achieving radial artery access are more than 95%.[27] Training programs are rapidly developing in both the United States and abroad. The Transradial Summit was held in Chicago in December of 2010, and the Transradial Interventional Program, sponsored by the Society for Cardiovascular Angiography and Interventions, was held in January 2011. Cardiology fellowships in the United States are beginning to incorporate radial training into their programs. Both the Transradial Intervention Course and Fellowship in India and the TransRadial workshop in France are 2 programs with international prestige.

Several complications are unique to the transradial approach. Spasm can occur with radial artery cannulation secondary to stimulation of alpha-receptors and the small size of artery. The majority of patients have severe and diffuse radial artery spasm that usually resolves spontaneously.[28] The use of sheaths with hydrophilic coating and the administration of intra-arterial antispasmodics like verapamil are helpful.[25] In addition, it is important to reduce patient anxiety and discomfort because this will exacerbate arterial vasoconstriction. Using smaller catheters and restricting catheter maneuvers are also important strategies.[28]

At the conclusion of a transradial procedure, sheath removal and radial artery closure must be accomplished in a safe and effective manner. Several devices have been developed specifically for this purpose. These include the TR Band (Terumo Medical Corporation, Somerset, NJ, USA), D-Stat Rad-Band with topical hemostat (Vascular Solutions, Inc., Minneapolis, MN, USA), and Radi-Stop (St. Jude Medical, St. Paul, MN, USA). A study by Rathore and colleagues of 790 patients randomly assigned to receive either the TR Band or Radi-Stop compression device after transradial coronary procedure showed that both devices were as safe and effective as hemostatic compression devices. However, more patients felt discomfort with the Radi-Stop device, and the time taken to achieve hemostasis was longer with TR band.[29] In the end, the choice of closure devices used will be up to the angiographer.

As the use of the transradial approach continues to expand, more research is needed to validate the safety and long-term benefits of this technique. The Radial vs. Femoral Access for Coronary Intervention study trial was completed in March 2011. More than 7000 patients were enrolled and the results were presented in April 2011 at the American College of Cardiology 60th Annual Scientific Session. The primary composite outcome of death, MI, stroke, and non-CABG major bleeding was similar between the 2 groups at 30 days.[30] It is hoped that more interventional cardiologists will adopt this technique as a viable alternative.

ANTIPLATELET THERAPY

The final event leading to ACS is spontaneous atherosclerotic plaque rupture. This event is similar to the "controlled injury" as described by Gruentzig during PCI. These events initiate a response that starts with platelet adhesion to the vessel wall, followed by platelet activation and aggregation.[31] The consequences of these processes are acute thrombosis leading to myocardial ischemia, infarction, and death. It is therefore of paramount importance to administer appropriate antiplatelet therapy during the peri-PCI period.

Antiplatelet agents have become the cornerstone of therapy in both ACS and PCI. Their efficacy has been well established in numerous large, randomized controlled clinical trials including Clopidogrel in Unstable Angina to Prevent Recurrent Events (CURE), Clopidogrel for High Atherothrombotic Risk and Ischemic Stabilization, Management, and Avoidance (CHARISMA), Clopidogrel and Metoprolol in Myocardial Infarction Trial (COMMIT), Clopidogrel for the Reduction of Events During Observation (CREDO), Trials to Assess Improvement in Therapeutic Outcomes by Optimizing Platelet Inhibition with Prasugrel–Thrombolysis in Myocardial Infarction (TRITON-TIMI 38), and Platelet Inhibition and Clinical Outcomes (PLATO). Furthermore, it has been well demonstrated that DAPT with both aspirin and a thienopyridine significantly decrease the morbidity and mortality associated with ACS.[32,33]

ANTIPLATELET MEDICATIONS

Aspirin, a cyclooxygenase-1 inhibitor, prevents the formation of thromboxane A2, a potent inducer of platelet aggregation. The Antithrombotic Trialists' Collaboration, which reviewed randomized trials designed to measure the effect of aspirin on outcomes, demonstrated a reduction in the risk of vascular events in all populations studied, including patients with prior or acute events and those considered at high risk of vascular events.[34,35]

The adenosine diphosphate (ADP) receptor antagonists are another class of antiplatelet agents that have played a pivotal role in the management of ACS. These drugs exert antiplatelet activity through action at the P2Y12 receptor. The P2Y12 receptor is found on the surface of platelets and selectively blocks ADP-induced platelet aggregation.[36] Three oral ADP receptor antagonists, ticlodipine (Ticlid), clopidogrel (Plavix), and prasugrel (Effient), are currently available in the United States. The action of these drugs is irreversible, meaning that the antiplatelet effect is sustained until platelet recovery. About 10% to 15% of platelets are replaced daily; therefore in approximately 7 days, platelets have returned to their functional state.[37]

Prasugrel received Food and Drug Administration (FDA) approval in July 2009 based on the landmark trial TRITON-TIMI 38. When compared with clopidogrel in patients undergoing PCI, this randomized controlled trial demonstrated a 19% relative risk reduction with the primary composite end point of death, nonfatal MI, or nonfatal stroke.[34] Two new antiplatelet medications, ticagrelor and elinogrel, are currently in clinical trials. A property that is unique to these 2 drugs is that they are reversible. These medications may have a compelling use in patients who may require invasive procedures or who develop bleeding complications while receiving antiplatelet therapy. Ticagrelor, which received marketing approval by the European Commission in December 2010 under the trade name Brilique, has a more rapid onset and more pronounced platelet inhibition than clopidogrel. The PLATO trial demonstrated a 16% decrease in rate of death from vascular causes, MI, or stroke in patients admitted with ACS, with or without ST elevation MI.[38] Of note, there was no increase in the rate of overall bleeding. Ticagrelor was expected to be approved in the United States in December 2010, but the FDA requested additional data analysis. Once approved, it will be marketed in the United States as Brilinta. Elinogrel is the only reversible ADP receptor antagonist available in both oral and intravenous forms. The availability of a reversible, intravenous ADP receptor antagonist could potentially be very beneficial to patients who have an acute need for antiplatelet therapy, or who are unable to metabolize medications via the gastrointestinal tract. Elinogrel, which has completed a phase II trial called INNOVATE PCI, showed a more rapid onset and great platelet inhibition when compared with clopidogrel.[39] A phase III pivotal trial is set to begin the first quarter of 2011.

CLOPIDOGREL HYPORESPONSIVENESS

Large clinical trials have shown that clopidogrel significantly reduces the risk of recurrent cardiovascular events in patients with coronary artery disease. Nevertheless, a wide individual variability in response to antiplatelet medications has been reported. In a meta-analysis of 14 studies with more than 4500 patients, 26% were classified as nonresponders and the remaining (74%) as responders.[40] Furthermore, there is an increasing amount of data on the relation between residual platelet reactivity and the increased risk of cardiac, cerebrovascular, and peripheral arterial events. In this study, nonresponders had a 5-fold increased risk of nonfatal and fatal cardiovascular recurrences than responders.[40] The clinical significance of clopidogrel nonresponsiveness is considerable.

Several pharmacokinetic and pharmacodynamic factors have been found to affect individual response to clopidogrel. Clopidogrel is a pro-drug that requires biotransformation to an active metabolite by cytochrome P-450 enzymes. The CYP2C19 gene plays an important role in the bioactivation process. Variants in CYP2C19, especially CYP2C19*2, are associated with variation in the bioavailability of the active metabolite of clopidogrel, and therefore alter the antiplatelet effect, and consequently, clinical outcomes. The incidence of carrying a reduced function CYP2C19*2 allele varies in the general population. Approximately 50% of Chinese, 34% of African Americans, 25% of whites, and 19% of Mexican Americans carry at least 1 copy.[41] Given the devastating outcomes associated with stent thrombosis and the prevalence of the CYP2C19*2 allele in the community, efforts are underway to determine individual responsiveness to antiplatelet therapy.

Responsiveness to antiplatelet therapy can be measured through several methods. These include multiple electrode platelet aggregometry, light transmission aggregometry (LTA), Plateletworks (Helena Laboratories, Beaumont, TX, USA), and through the use of a P2Y12 assay (VerifyNow, Accumetrics, San Diego, CA, USA) or a platelet-function analyzer. There is no uniform method, and therefore these tests may produce conflicting and ambiguous results, which may further cloud the clinical picture. The Do Platelet Function Assays Predict Clinical Outcomes in Clopidogrel-Pretreated Patients Undergoing Elective PCI trial was designed to help determine what method had the most predictive clinical value. The results showed that LTA, VerifyNow, and Plateletworks predicted adverse events associated with clopidogrel hyporesponsiveness[42]; however, the predictive value was modest. Based on these findings, the investigators could not recommend these tests to guide clinical practice. The Gauging Responsiveness with a VerifyNow Assay-Impact on Thrombosis And Safety trial is now underway to demonstrate the predictive value of the VerifyNow assay.

Another approach that is gaining momentum is testing for the CYP2C19*2 allele. Pharmacogenomics, a branch of pharmacology that deals with the influence of genetic variation on drug response in patients, is a growing field. Throughout the country, hospitals are offering genetic testing to determine individual response to many types of medications, including antiplatelet drugs. In September 2010, Vanderbilt Medical Center began testing all patients undergoing cardiac catheterization for genetic variations that could affect their response to clopidogrel. The intent of this program is help clinicians use appropriate antiplatelet therapy for each patient based on their genetic makeup, and to reduce the risk of future complications, including MI and sudden cardiac death.[43] As the public becomes more aware of this problem, there will be increasing demand for genetic testing both in the outpatient and inpatient arena.

Treating Hyporesponsiveness

When faced with clopidogrel hyporesponsiveness, there are several alternatives that should be considered in treating patients who require platelet inhibition. The American College of Cardiology Foundation/American Heart Association (ACCF/AHA) clinical alert published on August 3, 2010 provides evidence-based guidelines to aid the clinician in choosing an appropriate pharmacologic strategy.[41] Alternative clopidogrel dosing may be considered. This may include a higher maintenance dose of 150 mg daily (standard dose 75 mg daily) or a double loading dose of 300 mg. Prasugrel and ticagrelor are alternatives in patients with a known poor response to clopidogrel or in patients at high risk for a poor outcome from potential clopidogrel nonresponsiveness.[41] Adding a third antiplatelet drug like cilostazol may also increase the level of platelet inhibition. When using alternate dosing regimens or alternative drugs, additional testing may be needed to determine adequate platelet inhibition. More clinical research is needed to determine the safety and efficacy of each of these alternative regimens.

The Clopidogrel-Omeprazole Controversy

On January 26, 2009, the FDA published a warning regarding taking clopidogrel and omeprazole (Prilosec) together. They stated that "when clopidogrel and omeprazole are taken together, the effectiveness of clopidogrel is reduced. Patients at risk for heart attacks or strokes who use clopidogrel to prevent blood clots will not get the full effect of this medicine if they are also taking omeprazole."[44] The proposed mechanism of this reduced effect is inhibition of the CYP450 2C19–mediated metabolic bioactivation of clopidogrel by omeprazole. There was a strong reaction to this warning in the medical community because of the potential impact it would have on patients taking both medications. The medical community responded with a trial called Clopidogrel and the Optimization of Gastrointestinal Events, which was published in October 2010. In this trial 3800 patients were randomized to clopidogrel and omeprazole, or clopidogrel and placebo. The primary end point was bleeding or development of an ulcer. There was no difference in cardiovascular events between the 2 groups.[45] Despite these findings, the FDA has did not withdraw its warning. The ACCF/AHA stress the use of clinical judgment and weighing the benefits and risks of both cardiovascular events and gastrointestinal bleeding when placing a patient on concurrent therapy with both a proton pump inhibitor and clopidogrel.[41]

NEW THERAPIES FOR DYSLIPIDEMIA

High-density lipoprotein cholesterol (HDL-C) in plasma has been recognized as inversely related to the risk of developing CHD.[46] The Framingham Study showed HDL-C to be the strongest lipid risk factor compared with triglycerides, low-density lipoprotein cholesterol (LDL-C), and total cholesterol levels.[47] Each 1 mg/dL increase in HDL-C is associated with 2% to 3% decrease in the risk of CHD. Large randomized controlled trials using the current armamentarium of available medications have demonstrated that by increasing HDL-C, coronary events decrease. The Adult Treatment Panel III states that the major target of therapy in those with low HDL-C is LDL-C reduction.[48] However, analysis of statin trials demonstrates that despite LDL-C reduction, individuals with low HDL-C continue to be at risk. The development of new agents to raise HDL-C, therefore, is of great clinical importance.

The cholesteryl ester transfer protein (CETP) inhibitors are an exciting new class of drugs. These medications prevent transport of cholesterol from HDL to LDL particles, which result in an increase in HDL-C and a reduction in LDL-C. Torcetrapib, dalcetrapib, and anacetrapib are 3 CETP inhibitors that have been studied in clinical trials. The Investigation of Lipid Level Management to Understand Its Impact in Atherosclerotic Events trial demonstrated an impressive 72% increase in HDL-C with torcetrapib, but an increase in mortality and morbidity rates led to its discontinuation in 2006.[48] Since that time, both dalcetrapib and anacetrapib have been developed and continue to undergo clinical trials to establish safety and efficacy in high-risk patients. Dalcetrapib was shown in the DAL-Outcomes trial to increase HDL-C by 35% and importantly did not show any relevant differences versus placebo in adverse events. The DAL-HEART trial will look at how dalcetrapib affects the arterial wall and plaque in the coronary arteries.[49] The Determining the Efficacy and Tolerability of CETP Inhibition with Anacetrapib trial was established to test the safety of anacetrapib, the newest CETP inhibitor under investigation. After 24 weeks of treatment, there was 40% reduction in LDL-C and a staggering 138% increase in HDL-C cholesterol compared with placebo. There was no increase in the risk of cardiovascular events or mortality compared with placebo. The Randomized Evaluation of the Effects of Anacetrapib through Lipid-modification trial, which will determine the safety and efficacy of anacetrapib, will begin enrollment in 2011.[50]

SUMMARY

There are many new developments in both the invasive and noninvasive treatment of ACS. As technology, pharmaceuticals, and research continue to bring new therapies to the forefront, it is essential that clinicians stay current in their understanding of how this new knowledge will impact patients and alter clinical outcomes.

REFERENCES

1. Roger VL, Go AS, Lloyd-Jones DM, et al; on behalf of the American Heart Association Statistics Committee and Stroke Statistics Subcommittee. Heart disease and stroke statistics—2011 update: a report from the American Heart Association. Circulation 2011;123:e18–e209.
2. Mueller R, Sanborn T. The history of interventional cardiology: cardiac catheterization, angioplasty, and related interventions. Am Heart J 1995;129:146–72.
3. Grech E. ABC of interventional cardiology. Percutaneous coronary intervention. Br Med J 2003;326:1080–2.
4. Newsome L, Kutcher M, Royster R. Coronary artery stents: part I. Evolution of percutaneous coronary intervention. Anesth Analg 2008;107:552–69.
5. Regar E, Sianos G, Serruys PW. Stent development and local drug delivery. Br Med Bull 2001;59(1):227–48.
6. Okura H, Shimodozono S, Hayase M, et al. Impact of deep vessel wall injury and vessel stretching on subsequent arterial remodeling after balloon angioplasty: a serial intravascular ultrasound study. Am Heart J 2002;144(2):323–8.
7. Sigwart U, Mirkovitch V, Joffre F, et al. Intravascular stents to prevent occlusion and restenosis after transluminal angioplasty. N Engl J Med 1987;316:701–6.
8. Serruys P, De Jaegere P, Kiemeneij F, et al. A comparison of balloon-expandable-stent implantation with balloon angioplasty in patients with coronary artery disease. N Engl J Med 1994;331(8):489–95.
9. Fischman D, Leon M, Baim D, et al; Stent Restenosis Study Investigators. A randomized comparison of coronary-stent placement and balloon angioplasty in the treatment of coronary artery disease. N Engl J Med 1994;331:496–501.
10. Kotani J, Awata M, Nanto S, et al. Incomplete neointimal coverage of sirolimus-eleuting stents. angioscopic findings. J Am Coll Cardiol 2006;47:2108–11.
11. Rade JJ, Hogue CWJ. Noncardiac surgery for patients with coronary artery stents: timing is everything. Anesthesiology 2008;109(4):573–5.
12. Byrne RA, Mehilli J, Iijima R, et al. A polymer-free dual drug-eluting stent in patients with coronary artery disease: a randomized trial vs. polymer-based drug-eluting stents. Eur Heart J 2009;30(8):923–31.
13. Shand J, Menown I. Drug-eluting stents: the next generation. Interv Cardiol 2010;2(3): 341–50.
14. Doyle B, Holmes D. Next generation drug-eluting stents: focus on bioabsorbable platforms and polymers. Med Devices Evid Res 2009;2:47–55.
15. Han Y, Jing Q, Xu B, et al, for the CREATE (Multi-Center Registry of Excel Biodegradable Polymer Drug-Eluting Stents) Investigators. Safety and efficacy of biodegradable polymer-coated sirolimus-eluting stents in "real-world" practice: 18-month clinical and 9-month angiographic outcomes. J Am Coll Cardiol Interv 2009(2);303–9.
16. Garg S, Serruys P. Coronary stents: looking forward. J Am Coll Cardiol 2010;56: S43–78.
17. Fuchs S, Komowski R, Teplistsky I, et al. Major bleeding complicating contempary primary percutaneous coronary interventions-incidence, predictors, and prognostic implications. Cardiovasc Revasc Med 2009;10:88–93.

18. Yatskar L, Selzer F, Feit F, et al. Access site hematoma requiring blood transfusion predicts mortality in patients undergoing percutaneous coronary intervention: data from the national heart, lung, and blood institute dynamic registry. Catheter Cardiovasc Interv 2007;69(7):961–6.

19. Campeau L. Percutaneous radial artery approach for coronary angiography. Catheter Cardiovas Diagn 1989;16:3–7.

20. Vavalle J, Rao S. The impact of radial access on PCI complications: advantages of this approach in the outcomes of percutaneous coronary intervention. Cardiac Interv Today 2010:34–7.

21. Almany S, O'Neill W. Radial artery access for diagnostic and interventional procedures. 1999. Available at: http://www.accumedsystemsinc.com/resources/radial_artery_access_manual.pdf. Accessed January 25, 2011.

22. Hamel W. Fermoral artery closure after cardiac catheterization. Crit Care Nurse 2009;29:39–46.

23. Jolly S, Amlani S, Hamon M, et al. Radial versus femoral access for coronary angiography or intervention and the impact on major bleeding and ischemic events: a systematic review and meta-analysis of randomized trials. Am Heart J 2009; 157:132–40.

24. Kaiser C. Transradial approach gains momentum, and for good reason. 2010. Available at: http://www.cardiovascularbusiness.com/index.php?option=com_articles&article=20144. Accessed January 6, 2011.

25. Bilodeau M, Simon D. Transradial basics. Card Interv Today 2010:25–32.

26. Doganov A. The radial approach: en route to routine? EuroIntervention 2010;6:175–7.

27. Bertrand O, Mann T. Transradial approach for coronary angiography and intervention—ready for prime time? US Cardiol 2010;7(1):81–4.

28. Eltahawy E, Cooper C. Managing radial access vascular complications. Card Interv Today 2010:46–9.

29. Rathore S, Stables R, Maheshwar P, et al. A randomized comparison of TR Band and Radistop hemostatic compression devices after transradial coronary intervention. Catheter Cardiovasc Interv 2010;76:660–7.

30. SCAI Statement on "The Rival Trial: A Randomized Comparison of Radial Versus Femoral Access for Coronary Angiography or Intervention in Patients with Acute Coronary Syndromes." The Society for Cardiovascular Angiography and Intervention, April 4, 2011. Available at: http://www.scai.org/Press/detail.aspx?cid=10653c2b-e147-4a33-9788-1dee757de30f. Accessed April 28, 2011.

31. Alexander J. The current state of antiplatelet therapy in acute coronary syndromes: the data and the real world. Cleve Clin J Med 2009;76(Suppl 1):S16–22.

32. Yusuf S, Zhao F, Mehta SR, et al. Effects of clopidogrel in addition to aspirin in patients with acute coronary without ST-segment elevation. N Engl J Med 2001;345:494–502.

33. Wiviott S, Braunwald E, McCabe C. Prasugrel versus clopidogrel in patients with acute coronary syndromes. N Engl J Med 2007;357:2001–15.

34. Antithrombotic Trialists' Collaboration. Collaborative meta-analysis of randomized trials of antiplatelet therapy for prevention of death, myocardial infraction, and stroke in high risk patients. Br Med J 2002;324:71–86.

35. Alexander J. The current state of antiplatelet therapy in acute coronary syndromes: the data and the real world. Cleve Clin J Med 2009;76(Suppl 1):S16–S23.

36. Schindler C. New players in the field of antiplatelet and anticoagulant therapy in coronary heart disease—current therapeutic issues and hot topics. Ther Adv Cardiovasc Dis 2009;3(6):413–21.

37. Weber A, Braun M, Hohlfeld T, et al. Recovery of platelet function after discontinuation of clopidogrel treatment in healthy volunteers. J Clin Pharmacol 2001;52:333–6.
38. Wallentin L, Becker RC, Budaj A, et al. Ticagrelor versus clopidogrel in patients with acute coronary syndromes. N Engl J Med 2009;361(11):1045–57.
39. Rao S; INNOVATE PCI Investigators. A randomized, double-blind, active controlled trial to evaluate intravenous and oral PRT060128 (elinogrel), a selective and reversible P2Y12 receptor inhibitor vs clopidogrel as a novel antiplatelet therapy in patients undergoing nonurgent percutaneous coronary interventions. Available at: http://www.escardio.org/congresses/esc-2010/congress-reports/Pages/707-1-INNOVATE.aspx. Accessed September 21, 2011.
40. Sofi F, Marcucci R, Gori AM, et al. Clopidogrel non-responsiveness and risk of cardiovascular morbidity: an updated meta-analysis. Thromb Haemost 2010;103:841–8.
41. Holmes DR, Dehmer GJ, Kaul S, et al. ACCF/AHA clopidogrel clinical alert: approaches to the FDA "boxed warning": a report of the American College of Cardiology Foundation Task Force on Clinical Expert Consensus Documents and the American Heart Association. Circulation 2010;122:537–57.
42. van Werkum JW, Hackeng CM, de Korte FI, et al. Point-of-care platelet function testing in patients undergoing PCI: between a rock and a hard place. Neth Heart J 2007;15:299–305.
43. Vanderbilt Launches New Genetic Screening Program to Prevent Problems Associated with Plavix. Newswise, 2010. Available at: http://www.newswise.com/articles/view/568890?print-article. Accessed December 1, 2010.
44. FDA Alert. Early communication about an ongoing safety review of clopidogrel bisulfate (marketed as Plavix). 2009. Available at: http://www.fda.gov/Drugs/DrugSafety/PostmarketDrugSafetyInformationforPatientsandProviders/DrugSafetyInformationforHeathcareProfessionals/ucm079520.htm. Accessed January 20, 2011.
45. Bhatt DL, Cryer BL, Contant CF, et al. Clopidogrel with or without omeprazole in coronary artery disease. N Engl J Med 2010;363(20):1909–17.
46. Miyares M. Anacetrapib and dalcetrapib: two novel cholesteryl ester transfer protein inhibitors. Ann Pharmacother 2011;45(1):84–94.
47. Gordon T, Castelli WP, Hjortland MC, et al. High-density lipoprotein as a protective factor against coronary artery disease. The Framingham Study. Am J Med 1977;62:707–14.
48. Barter PJ, Caulfield M, LaRosa JC, et al. Effects of torcetrapib in patients at high risk for coronary events. N Engl J Med 2007;357:2109–22.
49. Executive Summary of the Third Report of the National Cholesterol Education Program (NCEP). J Am Med Assoc 2001;285:2486–97.
50. Olsson A. Novel CETP inhibitors in clinical development. Medscape Cardiology: Education 2010. Available at: http://www.theheart.org/documents/sitestructure/en/content/programs/1159377/Olsson.html. Accessed January 21, 2011.

Coronary Artery Bypass Surgery

Tabitha South, BSN, RN

KEYWORDS
- Coronary artery bypass graft • Open heart surgery
- On-pump surgery • Off-pump surgery • Alternative conduits
- Hybrid operating room

Coronary artery bypass graft (CABG) surgery has been a recognized standard of care for coronary revascularization of occluded vessels for a number of years, particularly for patients with three-vessel disease or left main coronary artery disease. Although there have been improvements in preventative care and education of the general population regarding reducing risk factors for coronary artery disease (CAD), it is still a looming diagnosis facing the general population. Although expansion and evolution of less invasive procedures such as angioplasty and stents have decreased the immediate need for surgery, many patients still require CABG surgery because coronary stenosis often reoccurs and less invasive options may not be applicable. Despite all of the improvements and innovations, CABG surgery still remains one of the most frequently performed surgical procedures in the United States.[1] CABG surgery has been shown to be more effective than other less invasive procedures for relief of recurrent angina and provides a greater expanse of time before symptoms reoccur and require additional interventions. As a result, it is imperative to have an increased awareness of surgical interventions, treatment options, and outcomes for patients undergoing this procedure.

The goal of the procedure is to revascularize and restore blood flow to an area of myocardium that is currently receiving minimal or no blood flow as well as prevent further cardiac muscle injury or death. During the procedure, a vessel is harvested from the individual's body (usually an internal mammary artery or saphenous vein) and utilized to bypass the area or areas of blockage within the coronary vessels (**Fig. 1**). Subsequently, the patient should experience a reduction in anginal symptoms, overall improved myocardial performance, and a better quality of life barring any major complications.

The author has nothing to disclose.
Critical Care Services, Baylor Regional Medical Center at Grapevine, Grapevine, TX 76051, USA
E-mail address: tabitha.south@baylorhealth.edu

Crit Care Nurs Clin N Am 23 (2011) 573–585
doi:10.1016/j.ccell.2011.08.011   ccnursing.theclinics.com
0899-5885/11/$ – see front matter © 2011 Elsevier Inc. All rights reserved.

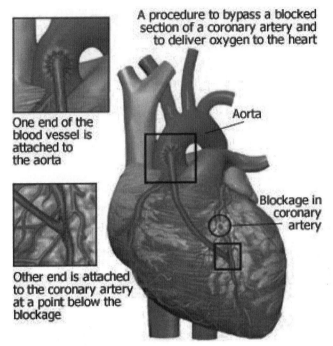

A procedure to bypass a blocked section of a coronary artery and to deliver oxygen to the heart

One end of the blood vessel is attached to the aorta

Aorta

Blockage in coronary artery

Other end is attached to the coronary artery at a point below the blockage

Fig. 1. Coronary artery bypass graft. Available at: http://www.heartonline.org/Coronary%20Bypass%20Surgery.htm. Accessed December 15, 2010.

OVERVIEW OF CABG SURGERY

Many factors are taken into consideration before a patient undergoes CABG surgery. Often patients may have had episodes of chest pain and a positive stress test followed by a cardiac catheterization to confirm the presence of CAD. During the procedure, stenotic areas of the coronary vessels are identified. Although many areas of stenosis can be treated effectively by percutaneous coronary intervention (PCI), there are some blockages that require surgical intervention. PCI includes procedures such as angioplasty, atherectomy, and deployment of stents. Interventional coronary procedures have significantly increased over the years as a result of gradually evolving technological advances, including the development of drug eluding stents. PCI procedures have been able to provide many patients with improved health outcomes while avoiding the need for cardiac surgery. However, when there are multiple diseased vessels with blockages, tortuosity, or an extensive myocardial infarction, surgery is almost always warranted.

CABG procedures may be elective, urgent, or emergent. In an elective procedure, the surgery is scheduled in advance. For example, the patient's coronary anatomy does not require immediate intervention and can be performed within a week or two. This may be the case when diagnostic angiography has been done and treatment is needed, but the patient is not actively experiencing symptoms. An urgent procedure occurs when the patient is in the hospital and symptomatic, or a significant stenotic area is identified during the cardiac catheterization indicating the need for intervention to prevent deterioration in the patient's condition. An example of this situation may be the identification of a 90% stenosis in the left anterior descending coronary artery.

Should the vessel completely occlude, a significant amount of myocardium would infarct. Emergent surgery occurs when there is a 99% lesion in the left main coronary artery, or after a mechanical complication of myocardial infarction such as a perforated intraventricular septum. In the urgent and emergent situations, patients are usually at higher risk for surgical and postoperative complications related to their declined state at the onset of the procedure.

THE SOCIETY OF THORACIC SURGEONS DATABASE PREDICTOR OF RISK

The Society of Thoracic Surgeons (STS) maintains one of the largest cardiac surgical databases in the world.[2] The database provides comparison data for facilities across the United States. It helps drive quality improvement initiatives that will further enhance cardiothoracic surgery outcomes. The data that are entered by clinicians across the world help to provide information regarding the impact of various risk factors on the outcomes of morbidity and mortality. At the end of 2009, there were more than 1000 United States hospitals submitting information into the registry.[2] The STS develops algorithms that are utilized to calculate a risk score based on specific pieces of information about patients such as ejection fraction, previous surgeries, diabetes, renal function, pulmonary function, and prior cerebrovascular accident. There are many more risk variables, but these are the more prominent variables that have an impact on the predicted risk calculation. Once the patient information has been entered, the clinician is provided a risk factor percentage that can be utilized to indicate if the patient is a low risk, high risk, or not a surgical candidate. Some institutions have guidelines using cutoff values for mortality and renal failure risk percentages to determine when a second surgical opinion or renal consult should be obtained.

USE OF CARDIOPULMONARY BYPASS

Isolated CABG surgery can be performed using cardiopulmonary bypass (CPB) or without the use of CPB. Those procedures performed with the patient on CBP are often referred to as "on-pump" while those that are done without CPB are referred to as "off-pump" CABG (OPCAB). The OPCAB procedure has often been described as "beating heart surgery." On-pump CABG surgery has been the standard for a number of years, but over the past couple of decades, there has been an increased interest in the feasibility of routinely performing off-pump CABG surgery. When CPB is being used, the heart and aorta are cannulated, the ascending aorta is cross clamped, and cardioplegic arrest is initiated. Complications may occur during the intraoperative phase of on-pump surgery, including "hemodilution, nonpulsatile arterial flow, global myocardial ischemia, atherosclerotic embolization from aortic manipulation, and systemic inflammatory response."[3] Complications related to on-pump surgery continue in the postoperative phase and have been found to lead to cardiac dysrhythmias, prolonged ventilation, cerebral dysfunction, hemodynamic instability, and myocardial depression.[4] Therefore, some clinicians propose OPCAB surgery would reduce the risks and complications such as systemic inflammatory response seen with on-pump surgery and the use of cardioplegia.

Patients typically require a vertical incision through the breastbone, and multiple blockages can be treated regardless if CPB is used or not although minimally invasive approaches may be used. Deep anesthesia is required for both. During on-pump surgery, the heart must be cooled and chilled, as the patient is placed on the heart–lung bypass machine. On-pump surgery is typically not performed on frail, elderly, or patients with kidney disease, lung disease, or those who are at high risk for complications such as stroke. In addition, hospital length of stay and recovery time postoperatively are often less for patients who undergo OPCAB procedures.

The touted outcomes associated with OPCAB procedures have been controversial when compared to the outcomes associated with the use of CPB. Therefore, several studies have been conducted to evaluate outcomes intraoperatively, immediately postoperatively, at 1 month, and at various timeframes for patients who have had both on-pump and off-pump cases. The following describes some of these studies.

The Randomized On/Off Bypass (ROOBY) trial was a large randomized study comparing the outcomes of on-pump versus off-pump CABGs. Almost 2000 patients were enrolled, with half of the patients undergoing on-pump procedures and the other half performed off-pump. Outcomes were evaluated at 30 days and at 1 year.[4] There were no significant differences in the outcomes at 30 days, but at 1 year, the off-pump patients had a worse outcome related to graft patency and less than complete revascularization.[4]

A retrospective analysis was completed by Mack and colleagues to evaluate on-pump versus off-pump surgery over a 3-year period.[5] The analysis included close to 2000 patients from four different centers that performed large volumes of heart surgery. The off-pump cases were found to have improved outcomes regarding morbidity and mortality.[5] The improvement was particularly noted in patients who were high-risk surgical candidates. An additional finding revealed CPB can be considered a risk factor for facilities utilizing off-pump CPB for the majority of the surgeries performed.[5] The investigators recommended that additional studies would need to be done to determine if the same is true if off-pump cases are a minority or nonexistent. The researchers attempted to evaluate outcomes beyond 1 year, but the sample size became smaller and not representative of the initial study sample.[5]

Brown and colleagues conducted a retrospective literature review finding mixed results regarding on-pump versus off-pump CABG procedures.[6] The investigators designed a study to determine which technique was best. Using an algorithm (**Fig. 2**) based on patient-related characteristics of coronary anatomy and comorbidities, patients were assigned to either the on-pump or the off-pump group based on the surgeon's evaluation of the patient. Patients with high comorbidities or found to be in the moderate risk group were selected for off-pump CABG.[6] It is important to note that only one surgeon performed off-pump procedure and the data from the 3 years of the study included only his patients. The main focus for this study was to evaluate the effectiveness of such an algorithm for determining the most appropriate type of surgical intervention. In the off-pump group, the patients were slightly older and had a STS higher predicted mortality than those in the on-pump group. At the 30-day mark, the mortality rate was lower than the predicted mortality in the off-pump cases.[6] However, additional comparisons, such as graft patency, were not made and long-term effects were not assessed. This study favored using off-pump as an option for surgeons for specific types of patients rather than looking at it as a competition between on-pump and off-pump surgery.[6]

Another area of research comparing the effects of on-pump versus off-pump CABG is neurologic compromise or changes. For years clinicians have thought patients who undergo on-pump surgery are at a greater risk for changes in cognition and motor abilities as well as an overall decline in neurologic function. These effects are sometimes referred to by bedside clinicians as "pump head." In the ROOBY trial, investigators compared the level of neurologic changes with on-pump CABG versus off-pump CABG. At the end of 1 year from surgery, almost 600 patients in each group underwent neuropsychological evaluation to assess for changes in cognitive status.

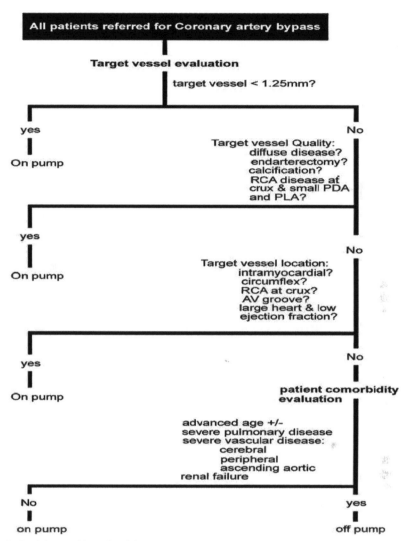

Fig. 2. Decision-making algorithm.

Results revealed there was no significant difference between patients in the on-pump group versus the patients in the off-pump group.[4] This result may be surprising to many. It may be beneficial to replicate this study. Dijk and colleagues also evaluated the neurologic status of CABG (on-pump vs off-pump) 5 years postoperatively in the Octopus Study.[7] This randomized control clinical trial was conducted for 2 years, enrolling nearly 300 patients. The patients in this study had undergone neuropsychological evaluation the day before surgery and 3 months, 1 year, and 5 years after surgery for the purpose of evaluating the effects of the two types of surgery on cognitive abilities. The findings revealed approximately half of each group had experienced some cognitive decline after 5 years. Neither technique was shown to be more beneficial for preventing a cognitive decline.[7] In addition, the researchers performed some evaluation of cardiovascular events postoperatively, finding there was no significant difference from one group to the other. In conclusion, the rationale that has been used to justify off-pump over on-pump because of perceived neurologic benefits appears to be unwarranted based on the results of these two studies. Completing additional studies on larger groups would be helpful in further validating these results.

Another area of controversy specific to on-pump cases is the effects of the type of cardioplegia utilized. Fan and coworkers conducted a meta-analysis evaluating the effects of warm versus cold cardioplegia utilized in on-pump bypass surgery.[8] The prevalence of myocardial infarction, postoperative length of stay, atrial fibrillation, and the incidence of intra-aortic balloon-pump (IABP) support postoperatively was the same in both groups.[8] However, the warm cardioplegia group fared slightly better in a few areas, including improved postoperative cardiac index and cardiac enzymes levels. Specifically troponin and creatine kinase-MB (CK-MB) were lower, suggesting that damage to the heart muscle may be somewhat less.[8] However, the overall results did not show a statistically significant difference to validate supporting the use of one type of cardioplegia over the other. The researchers suggested a next step to look at validating the decrease in damage and the impact it has on the recovery and well-being of the patients in a larger sample.

ALTERNATIVE CONDUITS IN CABG SURGERY

Conduits are the vessels that are utilized by a surgeon to bypass the blocked vessels within the heart. Each patient is evaluated to determine which conduit(s) will be utilized to provide the best graft patency and better outcomes long term. The surgeon evaluates patient characteristics, anatomical aspects, and available conduits coupled with surgeon expertise.[9] There are a number of conduits that are utilized including the greater saphenous vein (GSV); internal thoracic artery (ITA), also known as the internal mammary artery (IMA); and the radial artery (RA).

Conduit patency and long-term outcomes for patients are at the top of the list for surgeons when determining which conduit(s) will provide the best overall outcome for the patient. Conduit patency is affected somewhat by an individual's metabolic conditions, but based primarily on parameters such as ". . .degree of proximal coronary vessel stenosis, competitive flow from collateral vessels, poor distal runoff and size of the coronary target, conduit—coronary target size mismatch, site of proximal anastomosis and single or sequential type of coronary grafting."[10(p217)] All of these aforementioned factors affect vessel hemodynamics, blood flow, and stress to the vessel.[9] These can decrease the patency and flow throughout the vessel.[6] In addition, it is imperative to consider the circumstances that affect the graft directly. For example, when determining whether to use arterial or venous conduits, the surgeon takes into account that vein grafts have a higher rate of arteriosclerosis, and graft patency often begins to fail 5 to 10 years after surgery, while arterial vessels are more resistant to this.[11] However, arterial vessels also have their challenges. They are at risk for collapse and failure in the early phases if the need for graft blood flow is low related to a partial stenosis of the native vessel.[11] The options must be weighed using both patient and conduit characteristics.

The greater saphenous vein is harvested from the thigh or leg and is often used because of the ability to revascularize areas requiring differing lengths of vessels. Graft patency of the GSV is very high in the early periods after surgery.[9] About 50% remain patent 10 years after surgery due to arteriosclerosis.[9] One of the major issues with the saphenous vein is damage to the intima and cell wall related to techniques that are often utilized to harvest and transplant the vessel.[12] Souza and colleagues investigated the effects of harvesting techniques on graft patency of the saphenous vein in a randomized trial. They compared the traditional stripping method to a no-touch method and evaluated patency outcomes by way of angiography at 18 months and 8.5 years postoperatively. The no-touch technique involved isolating the vessel and a small amount of surrounding tissue to enable it to remain in situ for a longer period of time until extracorporeal circulation was initiated.[12] In contrast to the traditional harvesting technique, the vessel was not manually distended or stretched, nor was it flushed.[12] The study showed graft patency was much better when the vessel was harvested using the no-touch technique compared to the traditional harvesting process. They also found the better quality of the vein at the time of harvesting, the better the outcomes related to patency down the road. In addition, the investigators noted that a graft anastomosis also plays a role in maintaining patency. Grafts anastomosed distal to the sight of occlusion of the right coronary artery fared four times better when it comes to occlusion than those that were anastomosed above the crux region.[12]

The radial artery is another conduit that seems to be growing in favor. It is harvested from the forearm and can be removed because it is not the only source of flow to the hand. There are two arteries in the arm, the radial and the ulnar, and luckily, the ulnar supplies most of the blood to the hand, so patients do not often experience side effects from having the radial artery removed. The Allen test to determine radial artery patency is completed preoperatively and intraoperatively to determine if the radial artery should be utilized. The radial artery is a chosen conduit because it can be harvested easily, as well as its length and size.[10] The size of the radial artery is very similar to the size of the coronary vessels, which creates less turbulence of blood flow at the anastomotic site. Studies have shown that the radial artery is a great second choice as a conduit with the ITA being first. The ITA continues to be the gold standard for bypassing the left anterior descending artery, but the properties of the radial artery make it a viable choice for bypassing occlusions in other coronary vessels. Patients who undergo radial artery harvesting are given calcium channel blockers postoperatively to help avoid vasospasm of the artery.

The internal thoracic artery, also known as the internal mammary artery, is typically the chosen conduit because of its proven track record of survival and better patency. However, additional conduits have to be used because many patients have multivessel disease. One of the reasons this vessel is chosen is because it resists atherosclerosis development, contributing to longer graft patency.[11] In addition, the ITA is often able to be kept intact and sewn to the coronary artery just below the blockage because it has its own blood supply. If this conduit is not left attached to its normal location, and is removed for anastomoses, it is referred to as a free mammary artery. The ITA is typically anastomosed to the occluded left anterior descending (LAD) artery. However, trials have been done that have shown the left internal thoracic artery (LITA) grafts become occluded when the LAD artery stenosis is less than 70%, possibly due in part to a competition of flow between the native vessel and the graft, as mentioned previously.[11] **Fig. 3** indicates the common harvest sites for conduits.

Athanasiou and coworkers (2010) conducted a meta-analysis comparing patency and effectiveness of the saphenous vein and radial artery as conduits. The results were somewhat inconclusive at 1 year owing to variations in preoperative, intraoperative, and immediate postoperative management of the grafts as well as the patients' hemodynamic status. However, they found the radial artery is a superior conduit to the saphenous vein based on long-term graft patency of greater than 5 years.[10] Long-term patency is a better indicator of conduit graft effectiveness and atherosclerosis resistance.

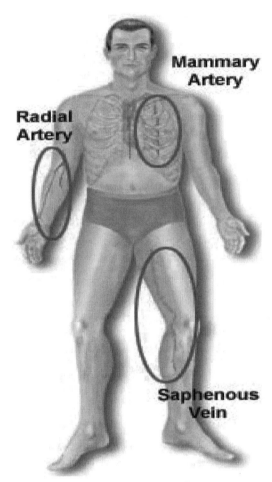

Fig. 3. Pictorial representation of typical conduits used for CABG surgery. Vessel harvesting. Available at: http://www.heartsurgery-hawaii.com/ vessel_harvesting.htm. Accessed December 15, 2010.

FUTURE OF CABG SURGERY
Minimally Invasive

Minimally invasive CABG is a relatively newer way to perform cardiac surgery without having to perform a sternotomy, and often without having to go on bypass. "Minimally invasive CABG is a surgical procedure based on the anatomic relations between the LITA, the coronary arteries and their branches, the apex of the heart, and the ascending aorta."[13] The surgeon must utilize criteria to determine if the patient is an appropriate candidate for this procedure. In addition to not using a sternotomy approach, the minimally invasive CABG differs from a traditional CABG in that single-lung ventilation is utilized. If there is a reason the patient would not tolerate single-lung ventilation, then he or she is not a candidate for this type of surgery. In addition, if the patient has disease of the ascending aorta or the subclavian artery, they are not ideal candidates for this approach.[13] It is also important to note that because this procedure is relatively new and specialized, not all surgeons have been trained in this approach, and additional considerations should be given to the experience level of the surgeon. This is especially true if the patient has had left-sided chest trauma that may alter the technique for surgery.[13]

Intraoperatively, the LITA is accessed through the use of electrocautery and anastomosed to the ascending aorta. An additional incision is made below the xiphoid process to allow for additional visualization and manipulation of the heart and surrounding vessels. A stabilizer is used to maintain the vessels location and anastomosis is completed.[13]

McGinn and coworkers conducted a study performing minimally invasive CABG in 450 patients in two different centers over a 3-year period.[13] Patients who needed emergent surgery or had severe pulmonary disease or severe pectus excavatum were excluded from the minimally invasive procedure. Instead of the sternotomy, a thoracotomy approach was used and the incision was made at the left fifth intercostal space and was usually 6 inches or less. Study results demonstrated minimally invasive CABG to be as effective in revascularization as a traditional CABG without an increased incidence of perioperative morbidity and mortality.[13]

Robotics have also contributed to minimally invasive surgeries becoming more prevalent, including heart surgery. Some trials have been done to evaluate the effectiveness and efficacy of robotics in heart surgery, with favorable results.[14] Endoscopic anastomoses of the LITA to the LAD artery has been done in various cardiac surgery centers across the United States and show favorable short-term outcomes without adverse events.[14]

Hybrid Operating Rooms

Hybrid operating rooms (ORs) are becoming more wide spread at various hospitals around the world. As minimally invasive, endoscopic procedures continue to grow, so will the need for hybrid ORs. They unite surgeons and interventional cardiologists with the focus on improved graft patency and long-term outcomes for patients.

In these high-tech ORs, imaging equipment is utilized to help take the guesswork out of determining patency of a potential conduit or blockages. Traditionally, surgeons typically rely on a transesophageal echocardiogram (TEE) to visualize the heart, but in a hybrid room, they get the best of both worlds with fluoroscopy and TEE. Some of the procedures being performed successfully in hybrid ORs include endovascular abdominal aortic aneurysm repair, select valve surgeries, and cardiac lead extraction. An additional advantage of the hybrid room is that if a case becomes more complex than expected or complications occur, it can be readily transitioned to a more traditional OR. Patients who undergo hybrid procedures often experience a shorter length of stay in the hospital owing to decreased overall recovery time and fewer complications such as bleeding and infection.[15]

Columbo and Latib reported results of a collaboration of surgeons and interventional cardiologists who utilized a hybrid room for almost 400 patients.[16] Before closing the chest, an angiogram was performed to evaluate for issues with a graft. If one was identified, an intervention was performed either percutaneously or surgically to correct the defect before the patient left the operating room. About 15% of these patients received a percutaneous intervention to correct a graft inadequacy.[16] Patients who underwent the percutaneous intervention in conjunction with CABG surgery experienced less time on bypass and less aortic cross clamp time. These patients also had a decreased length of stay and decreased ventilator time without an increase of blood product utilization. However, the downside to patients receiving an intraoperative percutaneous intervention was that levels of their cardiac enzymes, particularly troponin and CK-MB, were elevated, suggesting additional injury to cardiac muscle.[16] Some believe that using angiography in this setting may also help surgeons identify technique or graft selection errors that may lead to reduced initial graft patency. In this trial, there was a decrease in the percent of grafts that needed intervention as the team became more accustomed to the process in the hybrid room.[16]

Hybrid suites and cases continue to grow. In addition to CABGs with PCIs, valve surgeries are now being combined with PCI procedures. Complex aortic dissections and aneurysms are being treated with a combination of surgery and endovascular grafting.[16] Lastly, atrial fibrillation is being treated with a hybrid MAZE procedure.[14] The number of hybrid procedures are likely to continue to increase as technology and best practices prevail.

IMPLICATIONS FOR NURSING PRACTICE

The postoperative phase of cardiac surgery is very dynamic and challenges the bedside nurses to have a keen sense of monitoring and assessment skills combined with a strong knowledge base of cardiovascular care. On arrival to the intensive care unit (ICU), the patient is attached to monitors, allowing for continuous monitoring of hemodynamics. Blood work and chest radiographs are obtained shortly after arrival. The nurse caring for the patient postoperatively must monitor the hemodynamics, but also be cognizant of the patient's status. Close monitoring and management of the pulmonary status, bleeding, neurologic status, renal function, and pain control are also essential in the critical postoperative period.

The primary hemodynamics being monitored during this period include general vital signs, right atrial pressures (RAP), cardiac output/index, and stroke volume. It is imperative to maintain close control of blood pressure to help minimize added stress to the grafts and suture lines related to fluctuations in pressure or very high blood pressures. In addition, a patient who experiences hypotension will also have a decreased cardiac output, resulting in decreased perfusion of the vital organs. The pulmonary artery (PA) catheter provides important information regarding cardiac index, stroke volume, central venous pressure (CVP), and systemic vascular resistance as well as others to help provide a snapshot of how the heart is functioning and responding to surgery. These measurements help to provide a picture of the preload, afterload, and contractility of the heart and the effect each is having on compromising hemodynamic stability.

The heart rate and rhythm also require close monitoring, as there can be dysrhythmias that may occur postoperatively due to electrolyte imbalances including hypomagnesemia and hypokalemia, intraoperative myocardial ischemia, or myocardial infarction.[17] In addition, some patients require atrial or ventricular or dual chamber pacing and need to be monitored for complications related to pacing such as r on t phenomenon and failure to capture.

It is important for the nurse to have knowledge of the patient's preoperative pulmonary, neurologic, and renal status when evaluating the postoperative status. In addition, the nurse needs to know the effects of the intraoperative phase. For example, a patient who was in the operating room and under anesthesia for an extended period of time may take longer to regain pulmonary function and be weaned off of the ventilator.

Depending on the length of the procedure, prior respiratory status, and the surgeon and anesthesiologist's practice, the patient may be intubated or extubated on arrival to the ICU. The goal is to achieve early extubation because prolonged intubation can increase postoperative complications and may increase length of stay.[18] After surgery, a chest radiograph is usually completed and the nurse and respiratory therapist complete their assessments and follow-up evaluation of the lungs and oxygenation levels. The chest radiograph also helps to validate appropriate place-ment of lines and tubes and to confirm they have not been repositioned during transport. Arterial blood gases (ABGs) are usually obtained to assess oxygenation and ventilation status during breathing trials on the ventilator with the weaning process.

After surgery, some amount of bleeding is expected, but it should not be excessive. While the term excessive is objective, some clinicians consider chest tube output greater than 200 mL over 15 minutes during the first hour, but this should be clarified for each institution and surgeon. Hemoglobin and hematocrit levels are typically monitored using laboratory testing, but some facilities utilize some point-of-care testing to provide quicker results to the clinician. Some examples of point-of-care testing include point-of-care machines and noninvasive hemoglobin monitors. Some facilities utilize thromboelastography (TEG) to help evaluate clot strength and to help select appropriate blood products. A TEG can help provide information regarding which area of the clotting cycle is deficient to help the clinician determine if the patient needs platelets, cryoprecipitate, protamine, or other medications to help reduce bleeding. This test is particularly helpful when utilized appropriately by a trained clinician because there is justification for the type of blood product given. One of the goals of utilizing TEG is to decrease blood utilization while improving blood product management.

As mentioned earlier in the discussion, neurologic functioning and status is a concern postoperatively and can be affected by hypoxia, decreased cerebral perfu-sion, and embolism related to the surgical process.[17] Signs of postoperative neurologic impairment are most evident within the first 24 hours and should be monitored closely to prevent further decline or complications such as stroke.[17]

Renal function is also closely monitored to evaluate for complications related to comorbidities (renal insufficiency) or the effects of surgery and CPB. Frequent monitoring of urine output and trending is done along with monitoring serum creatinine levels. Patients are often diuresed postoperatively to help adjust for the fluid volume shift that occurs during and after surgery. When evaluating for appro-priate urine output, the nurse must also consider the effect of diuresis on the patient. One side effect of dieresis can be electrolyte imbalances, especially potassium depletion. Potassium levels should be monitored closely to help avoid dysrhythmias.

Another important aspect of postoperative care is adequate pain management. This includes providing education to the patient and family about realistic expecta-tions for pain after surgery as well as medication administration. Some patients expect to be pain free after surgery and are often surprised and upset when this expectation is not met. Communication and education regarding pain is important. If adequate pain control is not in place, the patient is not comfortable and is less likely to participate actively in his or her care to help prevent complications. This partici-pation includes being engaged in an aggressive pulmonary toilet and early ambulation to prevent respiratory complications. In addition, a patient's hemodynamic status is negatively affected by pain which further complicates the recovery process. In the initial postoperative period, pain is usually managed with intravenous administration of morphine sulfate, and the patient is transitioned to oral medications as tolerated to help prepare him or her for discharge and to prevent complications associated with intravenous narcotic administration.

A patient- and family-centered approach to care is ideal in the setting of cardiac surgery as well as acute care hospitalization in general. This approach includes the family as a part of the team that helps to prepare them to care for their loved one after discharge and to ease fear and anxiety for the patient and family.[19] Including families in the education regarding topics such as lifestyle modification, medication, and expected changes after surgery helps to prepare patients for going home and encourages an increased awareness of the expectations. This also provides additional support for patients as they transition into a changed lifestyle after surgery. Family members can also be involved in helping with activities such as pulmonary toilet and ambulation. Having them involved during the inpatient stage makes them more comfortable with helping their loved one and decreases the concern of hurting them if they move them the wrong way. Families are an important part of the care team and can help facilitate an easier transition from a critical patient to everyday life.

CARDIOVASCULAR SERVICE LINES

CABG surgery is also a profitable procedure in terms of reimbursement from insurers in comparison to many other procedures. This is one reason why many facilities have worked to build premiere cardiac surgery service lines. However, the additional costs that occur as a result, such as OR space and evolving technology, highly skilled physicians, and highly skilled nursing staff can often cause some facilities to evaluate their effectiveness and financial worthiness if they are a low-volume institution. Facilities that have large programs, close to 500 surgeries per year or more, have been found to have better quality outcomes and decreased mortality. This may be due to the fact that CABG surgery becomes more of a high-volume, low-risk procedure in comparison to facilities that perform fewer cases per year where maintaining top-quality metrics and knowledge base and skill set may be more difficult.[1]

SUMMARY

Coronary artery bypass surgery has taken many strides to become the effective intervention it is today. Although it has been the gold standard for cardiac revascularization for a number of years, the future of health care and technology will cause this standard to be morphed into a kinder, gentler approach that leads to even better quality outcomes and quality of life than is now expected. Research has been and will continue to be a focus in cardiovascular medicine and will only help further validate or dispute what is best for patients while challenging surgeons to become even more knowledgeable and skilled in the various treatment modalities. In addition, the emergence of super ORs will continue to blossom and create a highly technologically advanced environment that will limit the need for guesswork and gut feelings that many have practiced on for decades. The face of cardiac surgery will continue to change and we, as nurses, will be there to meet the challenge along the way.

REFERENCES

1. Wilson C, Fisher E, Welch G, et al. U.S. trends in CABG hospital volume: the effect of adding cardiac surgery programs. Health Aff 2007;26:162–8.
2. Jacobs J, Cerfolio R, Sade R. The ethics of transparency: publication of cardiothoracic surgical outcomes in the lay press. Ann Thorac Surg 2009;87:679–86.
3. LaPar D, Bhamidipati C, Reece T, et al. Is off-pump coronary artery bypass grafting superior to conventional bypass in octogenarians? J Thorac Cardiovasc Surg 2010; 141:81–90.
4. Shroyer A, Grover F, Hattler B, et al. On-pump versus off-pump coronary-artery bypass surgery. N Engl J Med 2009;361:1827–37.
5. Mack M, Pfister A, Bachand D, et al. Comparison of coronary bypass surgery with and without cardiopulmonary bypass in patients with multivessel disease. J Thorac Cardiovasc Surg 2004;127:167–73.

6. Brown J, Poston R, Gammie J, et al. Off-pump versus on-pimp coronary artery bypass grafting in consecutive patients: decision-making algorithm and outcomes. Ann Thorac Surg 2006;81:555–61.

7. Dijk D, Spoor M, Hijman R, et al. Cognitive and cardiac outcomes 5 years after off-pump vs on-pump coronary artery bypass graft surgery. JAMA 2007;297:701–8.

8. Fan Y, Zhang A, Xiao Y, et al. Warm versus cold cardioplegia for heart surgery: a meta-analysis. Eur J Cardiothorac Surg 2010;37:912–9.

9. Canver C. Conduit options in coronary artery bypass surgery. Chest 1995;198: 1150–5.

10. Athanasiou T, Saso S, Rao C, et al. Radial artery versus saphenous vein conduits for coronary artery bypass surgery: forty years of competition- which conduit offers better patency? A systematic review and meta-analysis. Eur J Cardiothorac Surg 2010; 40(1):208–20.

11. Sabik J, Blackstone E. Coronary artery bypass graft patency and competitive flow. JACC 2008;51:126–8.

12. Souza D, Johansson B, Bojo L, et al. Harvesting the saphenous vein with surrounding tissue for CABG provides long-term graft patency comparable to the left internal thoracic artery: results of a randomized longitudinal trial. J Thorac Cardiovasc Surg 2006;132:373–8.

13. Byrne J, Leacche M, Vaughn D, et al. Hybrid cardiovascular procedures. J Am Coll Cardiovasc Interven 2008;1:459–68.

14. McGinn J, Usman S, Lapierre H, et al. Minimally invasive coronary artery bypass grafting: dual-center experience in 450 consecutive patients. Circulation 2009;120: S78–S84.

15. Urbanowicz, J, Taylor G. Hybrid OR: is it in your future? Nurs Manage 2010;41:22–6.

16. Colombo A, Latib A. Surgeons and interventional cardiologists in a environment. JACC 2009;53:242–3.

17. Mullen-Fortino M, O'Brien N, Jones M. Critical care of a patient after CABG surgery. Nursing 2009 Crit Care 2009;4:46–53.

18. Martin C, Turkelson S. Nursing care of the patient undergoing coronary artery bypass grafting. JCN 2006;21:109–17.

19. Mullen-Fortino M, O'Brien N. Caring for a patient after coronary artery bypass graft surgery. Nursing 2008;38:46–52.

A Journey Through Heart Valve Surgery

Mallory Piaschyk, MSN, RN[a,*], Alaina M. Cyr, BSN, RN, CAPA, NE-BC[a,b],
Amy M. Wetzel, BSN, RN[a], Ani Tan, BSN, RN, CCRN[a],
Cecilia Mora, RN, CCRN[a], Doug W. Long, BSN, RN, CCRN[a],
Laarni Mendoza, BSN, RN, CCRN[a], Marivic A. Dela Cruz, BSN, RN[a],
Rebecca Gilliam, BSN, RN[a], Sheila Rolanda G. Bolanos, BSN, RN, CCRN[a],
Serena Stansbury, BSN, RN[a], Erika Diniz-Borkar, BSN, RN[a],
Charmaine Christiansen Moore, MBA/Mhsm, RN[a],
Lea Johanna Hyvarinen, BSN, RN[a], Catherine Fusilier, BSN, RN[a],
Natalie Culpepper, BSN, RN, CCRN[a], Suzanne Matson, RN, CCRN[a]

KEYWORDS
- Valve • Replacement • Heart • Graft • Surgery

The journey through heart valve surgery, related nursing implications, and patient education begins with an understanding of heart valves and methods of surgical treatment for insufficient valves (**Fig. 1**). There have been many advances over the past few decades in valve surgery since the first heart surgery was conducted on a young man in his early 20s in 1893 by Dr. Daniel Hale Williams.[1] Today, valvular heart disease is the fifth most common cardiovascular disease, with approximately 99,000 heart valve surgeries each year in the United States.[2] The necessities for valve surgeries are due to the incidence of valvular disease that occurs in individuals when valves are incapable of opening or closing sufficiently. The two main reasons that heart valve surgery is required are stenosis and regurgitation of valves. Stenosis occurs when the leaflets of the heart valve thicken, making it difficult for the blood to flow through the valve. Regurgitation occurs when the heart valves do not completely close, allowing blood to flow in the wrong direction. These processes interrupt the normal movement of blood through the heart's chambers and can cause a backup of blood in the lungs or the peripheral extremities, making it harder for the heart to pump the same amount of blood to the organs and the tissues.[3]

There are several alternative choices for treating valvular heart disease within our health care system today. Cardiac surgeons treat heart valve disease by either

[a] The Heart Hospital Baylor Plano, 1100 Allied Drive, Plano, TX, 75093, USA
[b] College of Nursing, University of Texas at Arlington, 411 South Nedderman Drive, Arlington, TX 76019, USA
* Corresponding author.
E-mail address: Mallory.piaschyk@baylorhealth.edu

Crit Care Nurs Clin N Am 23 (2011) 587–605
doi:10.1016/j.ccell.2011.08.006
0899-5885/11/$ – see front matter © 2011 Elsevier Inc. All rights reserved.

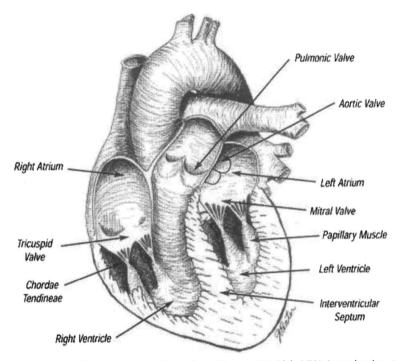

Fig. 1. Structures within the heart. (*Data from* Chung MK, Rich MW. Introduction to the cardiovascular system. Alcohol Health Res World 1990;14(4):269–76. *Photo courtesy of* Edwards Lifesciences, Irvine, CA.)

surgically replacing or repairing a dysfunctional heart valve or treating nonsurgically by monitoring a patient over time. Surgical methods to treat heart valve dysfunction or diseased heart valves are valve reconstruction, valve repair, and valve replacement performed with mechanical, biological, or homograft or autograft valves.[4] Valvular dysfunction can be either acquired or congenital, and it can affect people of all ages. Some factors that cause valvular disease are degenerative heart disease, rheumatic heart disease, and infective endocarditis.[2] It is crucial for health care providers to explain for each patient the rationale behind the type of surgery to be performed, discussing why there is a need to repair or replace the ineffective valve.

THE HEART VALVES

The heart valves determine the flow of blood through the heart. The valves open and close to allow for unidirectional blood flow, preventing regurgitation or blood flow in the wrong direction. Valves are classified as atrioventricular (AV) or semilunar. The two AV valves, the mitral valve and the tricuspid valve, lie between the atria and ventricles. AV valves prevent regurgitation back into the atrium during systole. The two semilunar valves are the aortic valve and the pulmonary valve. The semilunar valves are located at the base of the pulmonary artery and the aorta. These valves allow blood flow into the arteries and prevent regurgitation into the ventricle.[5–8]

Table 1 **NYHA classifications**	
Class I	• Cardiac disease
	• No limitation of physical activity
	• Ordinary physical activity does not cause undue fatigue, palpitation, dyspnea, or anginal pain
Class II	• Cardiac disease
	• Slight limitation of physical activity
	• Comfortable at rest
	• Ordinary physical activity causes fatigue, palpitation, dyspnea, or anginal pain
Class III	• Cardiac disease
	• Marked limitation of physical activity
	• Comfortable at rest
	• Less than ordinary physical activity causes fatigue, palpitation, dyspnea, or anginal pain
Class IV	• Cardiac disease
	• Any physical activity causes discomfort
	• Symptoms of heart failure or anginal syndrome may be present at rest

Data from American Heart Association. Available at: http://www.americanheart.org.

SIGNS AND SYMPTOMS OF VALVULAR HEART DISEASE

Patients with cardiac disease including valvular heart disease are classified using the New York Heart Association classification (**Table 1**) to determine the extent of disease.[9] Further, valvular heart disease can be classified into stenosis or insufficiency (regurgitation). In valvular stenosis, the stiff or fused valve leaflets narrow the opening of the valve. The narrowed opening can cause the heart to work harder, which can strain the heart and reduce cardiac output. Valvular insufficiency, regurgitation, or incompetence occurs when a valve does not close completely, causing blood to regurgitate back. The result is the heart must work harder to compensate for the incompetent valve, ultimately decreasing cardiac output.[8]

STENOSIS
Aortic Stenosis

Aortic stenosis (**Fig. 2**) is most commonly the result of calcification of a normal trileaflet or congenital bicuspid valve.[10] Aortic stenosis has the following classic symptoms: angina, effort syncope, and CHF. Studies have shown angina was seen in approximately 35% of patients, effort syncope in 15% of patients, and CHF in 50% of patients.[11,12] Angina is due to myocardial ischemia, which occurs when the left ventricular oxygen demand exceeds the left ventricular oxygen supply. Ventricular oxygen demand is the product of heart rate and heart wall stress. The compensatory mechanism to the pressure overload brought by aortic stenosis is left ventricular hypertrophy. The hypertrophy cannot cope with the pressure demands of the left ventricle, which in turn increases wall stress, causing an increase in left ventricular oxygen demand.

The syncope of aortic stenosis is related to exertion or exercise. The syncope is caused by inadequate cerebral perfusion caused by decreased cardiac output from the narrowed outflow tract, or by ventricular and supraventricular arrhythmias.[11,12]

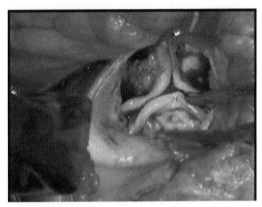

Fig. 2. Aortic stenosis. (*Courtesy of* Dr. Michael Mack.)

Another theory is that the peripheral vasodilatation caused by exercise in a patient with low cardiac output causes syncope.[12] Symptoms of CHF such as dyspnea on exertion, orthopnea, exercise intolerance, and paroxysmal nocturnal dyspnea are caused by left ventricular systolic failure and increased end diastolic pressure in aortic stenosis. In severe aortic stenosis, the high left-sided filling pressure leads to the development of pulmonary edema and right ventricular failure with symptoms of peripheral edema and ascites.[11,12]

Mitral Stenosis

Mitral stenosis is often caused by a mechanical obstruction of the inflow of blood.[9] The initial symptoms of mitral stenosis are exertional dyspnea, orthopnea, paroxysmal nocturnal dyspnea, and fatigue as a result of high left atrial pressure and increased pulmonary venous and arterial pressures. The increased left arterial pressure causes the left atrium to dilate and produce atrial fibrillation. Atrial fibrillation increases the amount of stagnant blood in the atrium, which can form a thrombus and enter the systemic circulation.[10] Atrial fibrillation and palpitations on exercise can also be considered early symptoms in patients with mitral stenosis.[12]

Tricuspid and Pulmonic Stenosis

Tricuspid stenosis symptoms include paroxysmal nocturnal dyspnea, jugular venous distention, fluid retention, and hepatomegaly due to right-sided heart failure.[12] Patients with tricuspid stenosis will often complain of fatigue due to low cardiac output produced by the narrow valve opening. Other signs of tricuspid stenosis are jugular venous distention, prominent A wave on central venous pressure (CVP) reading, and a diastolic murmur that increases with inspiration on auscultation of the left sternal border.[13]

Patients who have pulmonic stenosis are frequently asymptomatic and can tolerate moderate pulmonary stenosis (gradient <50 mm Hg) for years. Eventually, exertional dyspnea, chest pain, and fatigue can occur due to increased right ventricular pressure and reduced cardiac output. Signs of pulmonary stenosis include an obvious venous "A" wave in the neck and an ejection systolic murmur at the left second intercostal space heralded by an ejection or systolic click.[12,13]

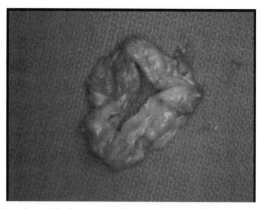

Fig. 3. Excised aortic valve with diagnosis of regurgitation. (*Courtesy of* Dr. Michael Mack.)

REGURGITATION

Aortic regurgitation (**Fig. 3**) produces symptoms of heart failure such as dyspnea on exertion, orthopnea, nocturnal dyspnea, and fatigue due to increasing left ventricular end-diastolic pressure, left ventricular dysfunction, and development of pulmonary venous hypertension.[12,14] Angina can also occur in aortic regurgitation because of an imbalance in coronary artery blood flow and left ventricular mass.[12]

Acute mitral regurgitation produces severe orthopnea or pulmonary edema due to failure of mitral valve leaflets to remain closed or rupture of the mitral chordae tendinae.[15] The characteristic feature of chronic mitral regurgitation is chronic volume overload.[16] The classic symptoms of chronic mitral regurgitation include dyspnea on exertion, which progresses to paroxysmal nocturnal dyspnea and orthopnea.[15,16] Other symptoms include fatigue, exercise intolerance, palpitations, and edema. Chronic mitral regurgitation can cause atrial fibrillation and palpitations due to increased left atrial pressure and left atrial dilatation.[15]

Tricuspid regurgitation is commonly attributed to either pulmonary hypertension or right ventricular dilatation associated with dilated cardiomyopathy.[12] Symptoms include fatigue, weight loss, cachexia, peripheral edema, ascites, hepatic congestion, and jugular venous distention.[17] The physical signs are large V waves on CVP tracing and holosystolic murmur along left sternal that increases with inspiration.[12,13]

Patients with pulmonic regurgitation are often asymptomatic unless right-sided heart failure occurs.[13] Symptoms include dyspnea on exertion, fatigue, light-headedness, peripheral edema, chest pain, palpitations, and syncope caused by right-sided heart failure.[18] Signs of pulmonic regurgitation reveal enlarged neck veins and other evidence of pulmonary hypertension. Also, a soft early diastolic murmur auscultated in the left upper parasternal region is characteristic of pulmonary regurgitation.[12]

DIAGNOSIS AND TESTING

Although the nature of the patient's heart valve disease can usually be ascertained from a thorough history and physical examination, diagnostic tests are essential to define the pathology and extent of heart valve disease more precisely. Both invasive and noninvasive modalities are available to obtain this information and should be chosen selectively. Various techniques may provide unique or complementary data, whereas others provide complementary information and need not be performed.

Chest Radiography

A two-view chest radiograph should be obtained on all patients before heart valve surgery. It provides ample information for compatibility with the diagnosis such as left ventricular enlargement in patients with volume overload (aortic insufficiency or mitral regurgitation), left ventricular hypertrophy in aortic stenosis, large left atrium in mitral valve disease, and calcified mitral valve annulus.

Electrocardiography

A 12-lead electrocardiogram can yield valuable information about the presence of atrial fibrillation and other rhythm disturbances. If sinus bradycardia is present, the patient will require temporary pacing postoperatively and may not tolerate beta blockers used prophylactically to prevent postoperative atrial fibrillation.

Myocardial Perfusion Imaging

Rest and stress imaging play a major role in identifying viable and ischemic myocardium. There are several forms of stress testing. In its simplest form, an exercise tolerance test is performed with a graded protocol on the treadmill.

Cardiac Catheterization

The gold standard for the diagnosis of most forms of valvular heart disease remains cardiac catheterization and is indicated in most patients for whom an interventional procedure is contemplated. The exceptions are acute type A aortic dissections and patients with aortic valve endocarditis and vegetations, in whom the risk of the catheter manipulation in the root is significant.

Echocardiography

Echocardiography is a valuable noninvasive means of evaluating ventricular and valvular function before, during, and after surgery. Although a transthoracic study is usually the initial study performed preoperatively, transesophageal echocardiography (TEE) provides superior imaging because of the proximity of the probe to the heart. TEE is very important in the preoperative evaluation of the patient as it provides a great deal of information, such as degree and nature of mitral regurgitation, mitral stenosis, aortic stenosis, degree of aortic regurgitation, and degree of tricuspid regurgitation.[19]

INDICATIONS FOR SURGICAL INTERVENTION
Aortic Stenosis

The degree of valve stenosis is used to determine the need for surgical intervention and is determined by measuring cardiac output (CO) and the peak or mean gradient across the valve (pressure obtained from the left ventricle or aorta). A valve area is calculated from the ratio of the cardiac output to the square root of the valve, known as the Gorlin formula (**Box 1**).

The average survival of the symptomatic patient with severe aortic stenosis is less than 2 to 3 years, and thus traditional indications for surgery have been the presence of angina, CHF, syncope, or resuscitation in an episode of sudden death. In contrast, surgery is usually not considered for the patient who is asymptomatic because the risk of sudden death is very low. However, the majority of patients with critical aortic stenosis will have symptoms in a short period of time and are at an increased risk of sudden death. Further, they can develop significant left ventricular hypertrophy (LVH), which is an adverse marker for long-term survival. Therefore, patients with severe or

| Box 1 |
| Calculation of valve area |

Aortic stenosis: calculation of valve area

$$AVA = \frac{CO/(SEP \times HR)}{44.5 \sqrt{\text{mean gradient}}}$$

where:

SEP is the systolic ejection period (per beat)

CO is cardiac output (mL/min)

HR is heart rate

AVA is the aortic valve area in cm^2 (normal is 2.5–3.5 cm^2)

Aortic stenosis grading:

Mild (AVA >1.5 cm^2)

Moderate (AVA = 1.0–1.5 cm^2)

Severe (AVA <1.0 cm^2)

Critical (AVA <0.75 cm^2)

Mitral stenosis: mitral valve area calculation

$$MVA = \frac{CP/(DFP \times FR)}{37.7 \sqrt{\text{mean gradient}}}$$

where:

DFP is the diastolic filling period/beat mean gradient

PCWP-LV is mean diastolic pressure

MVA is the mitral valve area in cm^2 (normal is 4–6 cm^2)

Data from Northwest Houston Heart Center. The structure of your heart. Available at: http://www.houstonheartcenter.com/html/heart_healthy.html; Bojar RM. Diagnostic techniques in cardiac surgery. In: Manual of perioperative care in adult cardiac surgery. Malden (MA): Blackwell; 2005. p. 61–81; and Choosing the right replacement heart valve. Harvard Heart Lett 2010;21(2):4–5.

critical stenosis require very careful monitoring for the development of symptoms and progression of valvular disease.[9,18,19]

Aortic Regurgitation

Surgical intervention is indicated for aortic regurgitation when acute aortic regurgitation is present with CHF. Other indications for surgical intervention include endocarditis with hemodynamic compromise, persistent bacteremia or sepsis, conduction abnormalities, recurrent systemic embolization from vegetations, or annulus abscess formation. The presence of symptoms is an indication for surgery as long as the aortic regurgitation is considered to be severe. If left ventricular (LV) function is normal (ejection fraction [EF] >50%), surgery is recommended for patients with a New York Heart Association (NYHA) class III–IV. If the EF is less than 50%, surgery is also recommended for patients in NYHA class II.[18,19]

Mitral Stenosis

The severity of mitral stenosis is determined by measuring the transvalvular gradient (pulmonary wedge pressure − LV mean diastolic pressure) and calculating the mitral valve area that relates the cardiac output to the gradient (see **Box 1**). Surgery is indicated in symptomatic class III–IV patients with a mitral valve area less than 1.5 cm^2, unfavorable valve morphology for percutaneous balloon mitral valvuloplasty (PBMV), left atrial thrombus, mitral regurgitation, or history of systemic thromboembolism from left atrial thrombus despite adequate anticoagulation. Generally, surgery is not indicated in patients with NYHA class I–II unless there is critical mitral stenosis (mitral valve area <1 cm^2) with severe pulmonary hypertension (pulmonary artery systolic pressure >60 mm Hg).[18,19]

Mitral Regurgitation

Surgery is indicated when the patient experiences acute mitral regurgitation (MR) associated with heart failure or cardiogenic shock, acute endocarditis with hemodynamic compromise, persistent bacteremia or sepsis, annular abscess, recent embolization for vegetations, or threatened embolization from large vegetations. Surgery is also indicated for patients with a NYHA class II–IV and severe symptoms. A symptomatic/class I patient should be considered for surgery severe MR is present.[18,19]

Tricuspid Valve Disease

A repair of tricuspid stenosis is indicated for class III–IV symptoms, including hepatic congestion, ascites, and peripheral edema that are refractory to salt restriction and diuretics. Repair of tricuspid regurgitation is indicated for severe symptoms or when moderate to severe functional tricuspid regurgitation is present at the time of left-sided valve surgery. Repair is especially important if the pulmonary vascular resistance is elevated. Severe tricuspid regurgitation is indicated if the mean pulmonary artery (PA) pressure is less than 60 mm Hg and if the patient is symptomatic after a trial of diuretic therapy. Surgery is a high risk for patients with a PA pressure that exceeds 60 mm Hg, especially in the absence of left-sided valvular disease. Surgery is also recommended for patients with persistent sepsis or recurrent pulmonary embolization from tricuspid valve vegetations.[20]

TYPES OF VALVES

Once the valve becomes ineffective to manage medically, it is imperative to look at the options for valve replacement if the valve cannot be repaired (**Figs. 4** and **5**). There are two options available for valve replacement, one of which is mechanical (**Fig. 6**) and is made of either plastic and metal or biological (**Fig. 7**), also called tissue or bioprosthetic made from harvested human donors or animals.[21]

There are many elements to consider when deciding what type of valve should be placed. If a patient is younger than early 60s and otherwise healthy, a mechanical valve is the better choice.[21] Mechanical replacement offers longer resilience and lowest likelihood of reoperation.[22] A mechanical valve can last 20 to 30 years or more and a biological valve can last up to 10 to 15 years. If the less than optimal replacement option is chosen, a replacement valve could wear out, requiring a second valve-replacement surgery. A biological valve may be a better fit for older patients or patients with life-shortening medical conditions.[21] The next factor to consider is anticoagulation. Mechanical valves are produced from artificial materials, therefore generating a life span of anticoagulation therapy for the patient is necessity.[23] Biological valves (see

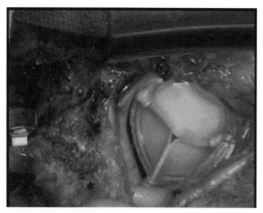

Fig. 4. Tissue valve replacement (*Courtesy of* Dr. Michael Mack.)

Fig. 6) are taken from human donors and or animals such as pigs and cows. Biological valves generally do not require the need for anticoagulation.[22] Another small but noticeable difference between mechanical and biological valves is sound. The biological valves will work silently, while the mechanical valve will make a quiet clicking noise that may be inconvenient for some.[21] Ultimately, the determination of valve replacement or repair is made on an individual basis.

DIFFERENT APPROACHES
Conventional Valve Surgery

Conventional valve surgery is still considered the gold standard for replacement or repair of a valve. During conventional surgery, the chest is opened by cutting through the sternum. This form of treatment, open-heart procedure, is performed under anesthesia with the assistance of a cardiopulmonary bypass machine.[24] During the repair or replacement of the valve, the heart is stopped using cardioplegia. Once this is done the cardiopulmonary bypass (CPB) machine is connected to the heart to divert blood from the surgical field. Once the valve is replaced or repaired the CPB machine

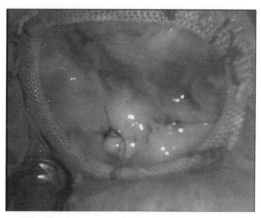

Fig. 5. Mitral valve repair with placement of valve ring. (*Courtesy of* Dr. Michael Mack.)

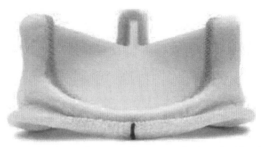

Fig. 6. Side view of tissue (biological) valve. (*Courtesy of* Edwards Lifesciences, Irvine, CA.)

is disconnected to allow blood to flow back through the heart. The heart is then restarted and inspected for leaking. These are relatively common procedures in cardiac surgery, but pose great risks to elderly patients.[24]

Minimally Invasive Port-Access Valve Surgery

Minimally invasive heart valve surgery or heart port procedure has been shown to be comparable to conventional surgery.[24] The port-access endovascular cardiopulmonary bypass is a closed chest endovascular system that enables aortic clamping, cardioplegic arrest, cardiac decompensation, and venting of the left side of the heart. The surgery is performed by making an incision in the right side of the chest between the midclavicular line and the right axillary line at approximately the fourth intercostal space. Cannulation of the heart to allow the use of the CPB machine is done through the femoral artery. The port-access is placed in the right internal jugular vein to allow for catheter access. Through the port and the incision in the chest catheters are used to manipulate the placement or repair of the valve. Cardioplegia is used to stop the heart. A video assist device is placed through a small incision at the second

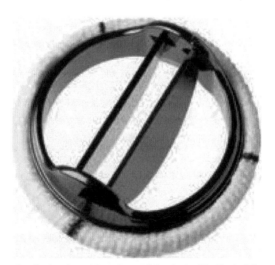

Fig. 7. St. Jude mechanical valve. (*Courtesy of* St. Jude Medical, Minneapolis, MN; with permission.)

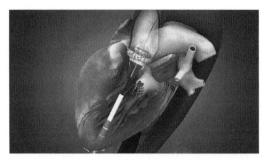

Fig. 8. Transapical approach to valve repair. (*Courtesy of* Edwards Lifesciences, Irvine, CA.)

intercostal space at the right midaxillary line. With the help of the video assist device and the transesophageal echocardiogram, the valve is repaired or replaced. This type of surgery has been shown to be successful; however, reoperation can be necessary at a later time.[25] This procedure cannot be performed on all patients, so selection must be done carefully based on age and the degree of valve damage.

Transcatheter Aortic Valve Replacement

The transcatheter approach to repairing the aortic valve is an emerging procedure that is considered palliative to provide temporary relief to a patient who is not a surgical candidate for conventional valve replacement. The procedure is performed by making an incision in the left anterolaterial intercostal to expose the left ventricular apex or transfemorally. When utilizing the transapical (**Fig. 8**) approach, a small puncture is made in the apex to allow a homeostatic sheath into the left ventricle. Transfemorally (**Fig. 9**) a sheath is inserted into one of the patient's groins, in which the valve is then replaced by having the sheath threaded to the left ventricle. The valve prosthesis (**Fig. 10**) is than crimped onto over a wire into the left ventricle. The placement is confirmed by echocardiography; rapid ventricular pacing is used to reduce cardiac output while the balloon is inflated, deploying the valve prosthesis within the annulus.[26] Reoperation from this procedure is very high, considering it is a temporary fix.

The Ross Procedure

The Ross procedure, first discovered by Donald Ross in 1967, offers a significant option for patients with aortic valve disease. The procedure is the replacement of the

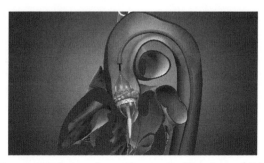

Fig. 9. Transcatheter approach to valve replacement. (*Courtesy of* Edwards Lifesciences, Irvine, CA.)

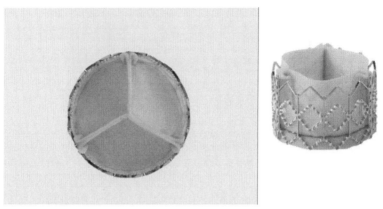

Fig. 10. Edwards SAPIEN transcatheter heart valve. (*Courtesy of* Edwards Lifesciences, Irvine, CA.)

aortic valve with the patient's own pulmonary valve, autograft, and then placement of a homograft in the pulmonary valve position. The procedure has since been modified from its original form to a full root replacement; which has shown a decreased need for reoperation. This option is favorable for a younger population and women of childbearing age because it eliminates the need for anticoagulation therapy, to allow the valve to grow with the patient, and has shown a low incidence of technical failure. Some contraindications include those with Marfan syndrome, active endocarditis, and an abnormal pulmonary valve. Overall studies support that a well performed Ross procedure can restore almost normal cardiac function.[27]

COMPLICATIONS ASSOCIATED WITH HEART VALVE SURGERY

Complications after surgery are atrial fibrillation, bleeding, infections, acute renal failure, respiratory failure, stroke, and systolic anterior motion experienced by patients undergoing mitral valve repair. Complications contribute to the increase in hospital length of stay as well as overall cost. The risk of complications increases with age, preexisting comorbidities, and the degree of disease to the valve.

Atrial Fibrillation

Atrial fibrillation (AFib) is one of the most frequent complications of cardiac surgery, affecting more than one third of patients. The development of postoperative AFib is associated with a higher risk of operative morbidity, prolonged hospitalization, and increased hospital cost compared with those in patients remaining in sinus rhythm.[28] The principal factor for AFib after cardiac surgery is increased age. Previous atrial fibrillation, mitral and aortic surgery, atrial enlargement, and withdrawal of beta blockers are also important risk factors. Other factors associated with development of AFib include the requirement for inotropes or vasopressors, hypomagnesemia, prolonged cardiopulmonary bypass, and impaired ventricular function.[29]

Bleeding

Major risk factors for postoperative bleeding are advanced age (>70 years), female gender, increased body size, CHF, and preoperative antithrombotic therapy. The major contributions to postoperative bleeding are inadequate surgical hemostasis, prolonged cardiopulmonary bypass time, hypothermia, residual heparin effect, platelet dysfunction, thrombocytopenia, and dilutional coagulopathy.[30]

Nosocomial Infections

Patients undergoing major heart surgery represent a special subpopulation at risk for nosocomial infections. Postoperative infection is the main noncardiac complication after major heart surgery and has been clearly related to increased morbidity, use of hospital resources, and mortality.[31] Cardiac surgery patients are at risk for three common nosocomial infections that include the lungs, the venous catheters and surgical site.[30] Also, cardiac surgery patients are at high risk for urinary tract infections.

Ventilator-Associated Pneumonia

Ventilator-associated pneumonia (VAP) is a severe complication after heart surgery. VAP is defined as pneumonia occurring more than 48 hours after initiation of mechanical ventilation. Although any patient with an endotracheal tube in place for more than 48 hours is at risk for VAP, certain patients are at higher risk. Risk factors that may increase the probability for VAP to occur include immunosuppression, chronic obstructive lung disease (COPD), and acute respiratory distress syndrome.[32] The goal is to extubate the patient within 4 to 6 hours after surgery if not sooner; however, underlying respiratory disease such as a history of COPD or smoking may cause a need to rest the patient's lungs or need for additional medication administration, extending ventilation hours postoperatively.

Postoperative Infection

The use of central venous catheters for vascular access and hemodynamic monitoring has become a central part of modern medicine. Although central venous catheters have significant benefits in many clinical situations, catheter-related infection (CRI) remains a leading cause of nosocomial infections, especially in intensive care units, and is associated with significant patient morbidity, mortality, and hospital costs. There are four potential sources for CRI: the skin insertion site, the catheter hub, hematogenous seeding from a distant infection, and contaminated infusate.[33] Maintaining aseptic technique with blood draws and dressing changes in conjunction with inspection of medications decreases the incidence of CRI.

Postoperative surgical site infections are a major cause of postoperative morbidity and mortality in cardiac surgery. A surgical site infection occurs when the contaminating pathogens overcome the host defense systems and an infectious process begins. Bacteria may enter the operating site either by direct contamination from the patient's skin or internal organs, through the hands and instruments of the surgical staff, or by bacteria-carrying particles that float around in the operating room and may land in the wound.[34]

Catheter-associated urinary tract infections (CAUTIs) are one of the most common types of nosocomial infection. Reducing the duration of catheterization is a key intervention in CAUTI prevention. For cardiac surgery patients, the recommendation for indwelling urinary catheter removal is 48 hours.[35]

Acute Renal Failure

Acute renal failure (ARF) develops in 30% of patients who undergo cardiac surgery and is associated with a high mortality rate (15%–30%). Several risk factors for ARF have been identified. Preoperative factors are strictly related to cardiovascular disease, advanced age, and baseline renal dysfunction, while intraoperative factors are linked with the type of cardiac surgery, the duration of cardiopulmonary bypass, and aortic cross-clamping.[36] Further, the single most significant risk for stroke is atherosclerosis of the ascending aorta. Other risk factors are vascular disease, advanced age, previous stroke, hypertension, diabetes, carotid artery stenosis, and peripheral vascular disease.[29]

Systolic Anterior Motion

After mitral valve repair, systolic anterior motion can develop. Systolic anterior motion involves prolapse of the anterior mitral leaflet into the left ventricular outflow tract (LVOT) during systole, causing outflow tract obstruction and mitral regurgitation.[29] LVOT obstruction due to systolic anterior motion occurs in 4% to 5% of patients after mitral valve repair. Systolic anterior motion after mitral valve repair can often be managed with beta-blockade and volume loading. However, the condition fails to resolve in some patients, who ultimately are better served with valve replacement.[37]

MEDICAL MANAGEMENT

In the decision to have valve surgery, the risks versus the benefits need to be at the forefront of the conversation with the patient, his or her family, and health care provider to make the best decision possible for that particular patient. Valve surgery has come a long way in prolonging quality of life. However, not all patients with failing aortic valves are candidates for open-heart surgery. Research suggests approximately one-third of the patients who could benefit from aortic valve replacement do not or never undergo the surgery.[3] In most cases, these patients are ruled out because of their higher surgical risk level.

Some options other than open-heart valve surgery for patients include but are not limited to balloon aortic valvuloplasty, transcatheter aortic valve implantation, laser angioplasty, and valvular clips.

Recovering from Valve Surgery

After valvular surgery, the patient is admitted into an intensive care setting to begin the recovery process. Within a few hours, the patient begins to wake up from anesthesia and the nurse assesses the patient's neurologic status. When the patient is completely awake and following commands, the patient is extubated while maintaining oxygenation. Oxygen will then be delivered through a facemask to nasal cannula depending on the patient's oxygen saturation and respiratory effort, with the goal of eventually weaning completely off as the recovery progresses.

Several types of tubes may be inserted to drain excess fluids during the recovery period. Chest tubes are inserted into the chest near the heart and lungs to drain the extra air and fluids that collect in the chest cavity during the surgery. The tubes are removed when the drainage decreases.

There are several intravenous (IV) lines in the arms and neck for monitoring of vital signs, administering medication, drawing blood, and replacing the fluids and blood lost during surgery. Pulmonary artery catheter or Swan-Ganz is inserted and is used to measure heart function and pressure in the heart. Readings from this catheter are used to adjust medications and IV fluids. An arterial line is placed in the artery of the arm or leg to measure blood pressure more accurately and may also assist in drawing blood.

EKG monitoring is tracked from the time the patient leaves the operating room until discharge from the hospital, which allows trending the patient's condition. Temporary pacemaker wires are placed intraoperatively to allow the heart to be paced at a controlled rate. Pacemaker wires are removed before the patient goes home; however, some patients may require the placement of a pacemaker before the pacemaker wires are removed owing to the patient's intrinsic heart rate not returning after surgery.

After about 24 hours in the intensive care setting, the patient is usually transferred to a step-down unit or to a step-down status, where the recovery continues. The patient will have an incision on the chest that goes from the top of the sternum to the bottom of the sternum, or alternative incisions around the side of the chest depending on the type of approach utilized by the surgeon. Pain, muscle aches, and soreness at the incision sites are normal as a result of the incisions themselves and positioning in the operating room. One major reduction of the incisional pain can be assisted by a pillow being held against the chest for splinting such as coughing or repositioning.

Breathing treatments or drug aerosol treatments are administered several times a day to loosen the mucus in the lungs, allowing the patient to breathe more deeply. The frequency of treatment will decrease as the lungs improve. The patient will use an incentive spirometer to help exercise the lungs, thus preventing complications such as atelectasis. Breathing deeply and coughing 10 to 20 times every hour helps keep lungs working well. It is important to instruct the patient to continue deep breathing and coughing exercises after he or she is discharged home.

Nutrition needs to be maintained in the recovery period. Patients are started on ice chips once extubated and then clear liquid are started when the patient has bowel sounds. A normal diet is resumed once a liquid diet is tolerated.

As tubes and IV lines are removed, activity is increased. Activity is started about 4 hours after extubation. Leg exercises are done while the patient is resting in the bed; activities such as pointing and flexing the feet and toes improve the blood flow to and from the legs and start the idea of getting mobilized. These exercises decrease swelling, prevent blood clot formation, and reduce leg pain. Sitting at the edge of the bed and then moving to the chair is the first step in increased activity. The importance of an ambulation program is imperative to the recovery process. Walking length, frequency, and time are gradually increased each day until discharge, while during this time physical therapy and cardiac rehabilitation personnel will be assessing for further needs. It is important to watch the patient for signs and symptoms of chest pain, dizziness, or shortness of breath.

Discharge teaching is started from the first day of hospitalization to prepare the patient and caregivers to go from the hospital to the home. Patients usually have 4- to 5-day hospital stays unless complications occur. During the first to second week after being discharged from the hospital, the patient should have 24-hour support at home. Some patients may need home health care after the surgery. The incision should be checked each time a patient bathes. It is normal to see clear, watery, pink, or reddish drainage on the chest incision for the first few days. The incision should be washed gently with soap and water each day. Showers should not be longer than 10 minutes, and extreme water temperatures should be avoided. Rubbing the incision with a washcloth should be avoided until the wound is healed and a scab forms. Ointments, salves, oils, or dressings should not be applied unless directed by the physician. If legs become swollen, elevating the legs above the heart level when resting and wearing support hose could be helpful. Prescribed medications should be taken as directed. Stool softener is given to decrease constipation from pain medication. Prescription pain pills may be taken for 2 to 8 weeks after surgery. Daily weight should be taken at the same time each day with the patient wearing the same amount of clothing. During the 6- to 8-week healing period, light household chores may be done; however, standing in one place for longer than 15 minutes should be

602 Piaschyk et al

Box 2
Signs and symptoms for which to call physician

Patients should be instructed to call the physician doctor if any of the following occur:

- Signs of infection, including fever of 101°F or higher and chills
- Redness, swelling, increasing pain, excessive bleeding, or discharge from the incision site
- Breastbone feels like it moves or it pops or cracks
- Nausea or vomiting that cannot be controlled with the medicines given after surgery or that persists for >2 days after discharge from the hospital
- Pain that cannot be controlled with pain medication
- Cough, shortness of breath not relieved by rest or felling faint
- Weight gain of 3–5 lbs or more in <1 week
- Rapid heart rate
- Pain, burning, urgency, frequency of urination, or persistent bleeding in the urine or unable to urinate

Data from Cedars-Sinai. Heart valve repair and replacement. Available at: http://www.cedars-sinai.edu/Patients/Programs-and-Services/Heart-Institute/Cardiothoracic-Surgery-Services/Heart-Valve-Repair-and-Replacement; and Todd BA, Higgins K. Recognizing aortic and mitral valve disease. Nursing 2005;35(6):58–64.

---

avoided. Lifting, pushing, or pulling objects greater than 5 to 10 lbs should be avoided. Climbing stairs should be avoided the first few weeks after surgery. Patients should rest between activities.

Patients can ride as passengers in a car, but driving should be avoided for 4 to 6 weeks. Breathing exercises such as incentive spirometry should still be continued for 4 to 6 weeks after surgery. If oxygen is needed, home arrangements will be made before the patient leaves the hospital.

Cardiac rehabilitation programs combine education, risk factor modification, and exercise to improve the patient's physiologic, psychological, and vocational status, thus preventing the underlying disease from progressing. It is divided into four phases: phase 1, hospitalization or inpatient, which lasts throughout the hospital stay; phase 2, early recovery or outpatient, which lasts 2 to 12 weeks; phase 3, late recovery, which lasts 6 to 12 months; and phase 4, the maintenance phase, which is self directed and lifelong.

Sexual activity usually resumes after 6 to 8 weeks when the sternum heals. If the patient can climb two flights of stairs or walk briskly for three blocks, then he or she is ready to resume sexual activity. It should be progressed gradually, assuming the nondominant role for a period of time. Sex should be stopped if chest pain, unusual shortness of breath, or irregular heartbeat occurs.

Returning to work depends on the degree of damage to the heart, the rate of recovery, and the job's physical requirements. Patients with a sedentary job could return to work in 1 to 2 months. Those who have more physically intensive jobs should resume their job functions slowly. Some may need to find another job that is less physical.

Patients also need specific information on when to call their physician. **Box 2** provides a list of situations for which the patient should notify his or her health care provider.

Lifestyle Changes

After heart valve surgery, lifestyle changes are required to maximize and maintain the new valve, as well as the overall health of the patient. Immediately after open heart surgery, which is most often required for valve replacement, sternal precautions must be taken. Sternal precautions include crossing arms across the chest when coughing, holding arms close to the body with weight-bearing activities (up to 8 weeks postoperatively), log-rolling to get in and out of bed, and moving arms only within a pain-free range.[38,39] Follow-up appointments must be kept with cardiologists, cardiothoracic surgeons, and any other physicians managing the care of the patient. On discharge, patients will be given a time frame for follow-up appointments and contact information for each specific physician. Patients should attend cardiac rehabilitation, beginning approximately 6 to 8 weeks postoperatively. Patients should be prepared to adopt a daily routine of weighing themselves and keeping an accurate record of daily weights. Patients should report a sudden weight gain to their cardiologist. This could be an indication of an inadequate valve. Valve replacement patients will require specific lifestyle changes associated with anticoagulation therapy to prevent thrombosis. Patients taking oral anticoagulants should be aware of possible food and drug interactions that can alter coagulation. Patients who are beginning anticoagulation therapy for the first time should receive both pharmacist and nutritionist consults. Patients should also be told what specific international normalized ration (INR) level is optimal for them, and be prepared for frequent blood draws at follow-up doctor appointments to monitor INR levels. For prosthetic valve patients, anticoagulation is lifelong therapy. Patients should also take special precautions to prevent the development of endocarditis. This includes informing all health care providers about the history of valve surgery. In addition, there is a lifelong requirement for antibiotic prophylaxis for dental, endoscopic, and surgical procedures.[40] A heart-healthy diet is recommended for all patients after heart surgery, including valve replacement patients. A diet with a variety of fruits and vegetables, whole grains, lean meats, low sodium, and low fat is recommended.[41]

SUMMARY

It is evident that valvular surgeries have made countless advances since the first valve surgery in 1925 when Dr Henry Souttar operated on a woman with mitral stenosis.[42] Patients in the 21st century have a better chance of surviving as a result of these advances. In addition to providing high-quality health care to patients, educating patients and their families regarding the disease processes, symptoms, diagnosis, types of valve surgeries, different approaches, complications, nonsurgical care, recovery, and lifestyle changes is an instrumental component to a successful recovery.

REFERENCES

1. Williams DH. Stab wound of the heart, pericardium—suture of the pericardium—recovery—patient alive three years afterward. Med Rec 1897;1–8.
2. Wiegand DL. Advances in cardiac surgery: valve repair. Crit Care Nurse 2003;23(2):72.
3. University of Southern California, Department of Cardiothoracic Surgery. Mitral valve repair. 27 Dec. 2010. Available at: http://www.cts.usc.edu/mitralvalverepair.html. Accessed December 27, 2010.
4. Cedars-Sinai. Heart valve repair and replacement. Available at: http://www.cedars-sinai.edu/Patients/Programs-and-Services/Heart-Institute/Cardiothoracic-Surgery-Services/Heart-Valve-Repair-and-Replacement. Accessed December 28, 2010.

5. Heart Information Center. Heart anatomy. Available at: http://www.texasheartinstitute. org/HIC/Anatomy/anatomy2.cfm. Accessed December 28, 2010.

6. Chung MK, Rich MW. Introduction to the cardiovascular system. Alcohol Health Res World 1990;14(4):269–76.

7. Northwest Houston Heart Center. The structure of your heart. Available at: http:// www.houstonheartcenter.com/html/heart_healthy.html. Accessed December 28, 2010.

8. Cleveland Clinic. Types of valve diseases. 28 Dec. 2010 Available at: http://www. my.cleveland.org/heart/disorders/valve/valve_types.aspx. Accessed December 28, 2010.

9. American Heart Association. Available at: http://www.americanheart.org. Accessed March 18, 2011.

10. Carabello BA, Crawford MH. Aortic stenosis. In: Crawford MH. Current diagnosis & treatment in cardiology. 3rd edition. New York: Lange Medical Books; 2009. p. 108–20.

11. Henein M. Heart valve disease. In: Warrell DA, Cox TM, Firth JD, Ogg GS, editors. Oxford textbook of medicine. 5th edition. New York: Oxford University Press; 2010.

12. Hoit BD, Varahan SL. In: Crawford MH. Current diagnosis & treatment in cardiology. 3rd edition. New York: Lange Medical Books; 2009. p. 151–66.

13. Maganti K, Rigolin VH, Sarano ME, Bonow RO. Valvular heart disease: diagnosis and management. Mayo Clinic Proc 2010;5(5):483–500.

14. Crawford MH. Mitral regurgitation. In: Crawford MH. Current diagnosis & treatment in cardiology. 3rd edition. New York: Lange Medical Books; 142–50.

15. Todd BA, Higgins K. Recognizing aortic and mitral valve disease. Nursing 2005;35(6): 58–64.

16. Diepenbrock NH. Quick reference to critical care. Philadelphia: Lippincott; 1999.

17. Ren XM, Cannistra LB. Pulmonic regurgitation. Available at: http://emedicine. medscape.com/article/157639-overview. Accessed August 5, 2010.

18. Bojar RM. Diagnostic techniques in cardiac surgery. In: Manual of perioperative care in adult cardiac surgery. Malden (MA): Blackwell; 2005. p. 61–81.

19. Bojar RM. Synopsis of adult cardiac surgical disease. In: Manual of perioperative care in adult cardiac surgery. Malden (MA): Blackwell; 2005. p. 14–29.

20. Choosing the right replacement heart valve. Harvard Heart Lett 2010;21(2):4–5.

21. A Patient's Guide to Heart Surgery. Heart valve surgery. Available at: http://www. cts.usc.edu/hpg-heartvalvesurgery.html. Accessed December 10, 2010.

22. Kark VA. What's new in cardiac surgery? Transapical valves. OR Nurs 2010; A Patient's Guide to Heart Surgery 4(5):26–34.

23. Conn L. Valve surgery options. In: Proceedings of the NHLBI Conference: Cardiovascular Health and Disease in Women: "Valvular Heart Disease." Baltimore: Le Jacq Communication Publishing Company; 1983. p. 335–9.

24. Mohr FW, Falk V, Diegeler A, et al. Minimally invasive port-access mitral valve surgery. J Thorac Cardiovasc Surg 1998;115(3):567–76.

25. Lichtenstein SV, Cheung A, Ye J, et al. Transapical transcatheter aortic valve implantation in humans: initial clinical experience. Circulation 2006;114(6):591–6.

26. Stelzer P, Weinrauch S, Tranbaugh R. Ten years of experience with the modified ross procedure. J Thorac Cardiovasc Surg 1998;115(5):1091–5.

27. Hogue CJ, Creswell LL, Gutterman DD, Fleisher LA. Epidemiology, mechanisms, and risks: American College of Chest Physicians guidelines for the prevention and management of postoperative atrial fibrillation after cardiac surgery. Chest 2005;128(2): s9–s16.

28. Sidebtoham D, McKee A, Gillham M, et al. Cardiothoracic Critical Care. Philadelphia: Elsevier; 2007. p. 158–73.
29. Ferraris VA, Spiess BD. Perioperative blood transfusion and blood conservation in cardiac surgery: the Society of Thoracic Surgeons and the Society of Cardiovascular Anesthesiologists Clinical Practice Guideline 2007. Ann Thorac Surg 2007;85(5): 27–86.
30. Hortal J, Muñoz P, Cuerpo G, et al. Ventilator-associated pneumonia in patients undergoing major heart surgery: an incidence study in Europe. Crit Care 2009;13(3): R80.
31. Augustyn B. Ventilator-associated pneumonia: risk factors and prevention. Crit Care Nurs 2007;27(4):32.
32. Öncü S, Sakarya S. Central venous catheter-related infections: an overview with special emphasis on diagnosis, prevention and management. Internet J Anesth 2003;7(1):16.
33. Gårdlund B. Postoperative surgical site infections in cardiac surgery—an overview of preventive measures. Acta Pathol Microbiol Immunol Scand 2007;115(9):989–95.
34. Saint S. State of the science: clinical and economic consequences of nosocomial catheter-related bacteriuria. Am J Infect Control 2000;28(1):68–75.
35. Morabito S, Guzzo I, Solazzo A, et al. Acute renal failure following cardiac surgery. G Ital Nefrol 2007;24(6):628–9.
36. Leonid S, Zehr KJ. Systolic anterior motion of the mitral valve after mitral valve repair: a method of prevention. Tex Heart Inst J 2005;32(1):47–9.
37. Lung B, Baron G, Butchart EG, et al. A prospective survey of patients with valvular disease in Europe: the Euro Heart Survey on Valvular Heart Disease. Eur Heart J 2003;24:1231–43.
38. Brocki BC, Thorup CB, Andreasen JJ. Precautions related to midline sternotomy in cardiac surgery: a review of mechanical stress factors leading to sternal complications. Eur J Cardiovasc Nurs 2010;9(2):7–84.
39. Butchart E, Gohlke-Barwolf C, Antunes M, et al. Recommendations for the management of patients after heart valve surgery. Eur Heart J 2005;26:2463–71.
40. Lichtenstein AH, Appel LJ, Brands M, et al. Diet and lifestyle recommendations revision 2006: a Scientific Statement from the American Heart Association Nutrition Committee. Circulation 2006;114(1):82–96.
41. Souttar HS. The surgical treatment of mitral stenosis. Br Med J 1925;2:603–6.
42. Baylor Health Care System. Patient discharge instructions. Dallas (TX): Baylor Health Care System; 2010.

Cardiogenic Shock

Margaret E. McAtee, MN, RN, ACNP-BC, CCRN

KEYWORDS

- Cardiogenic shock • Shock • Acute myocardial infarction
- ST elevation MI • Treatment guidelines

Treatment for patients with an acute myocardial infarction (AMI) has changed dramatically over the past few decades. Despite these advances, for the 5% to 10% of AMI patients who develop cardiogenic shock, the prognosis is very poor. Although the mortality rate has declined, it still remains at approximately 50%.[1–3] If renal failure develops, the survival rate is reduced further by an additional 20%.[4] This article provides a review of the current understanding of the etiologies, pathophysiology, and recommendations for management of cardiogenic shock.

DEFINITION

Cardiogenic shock can be defined as a decrease in cardiac output (CO) with evidence of tissue hypoperfusion, in the presence of adequate circulating blood volume.[2] The hemodynamic criteria include sustained hypotension, meaning a systolic blood pressure less than 90 mm Hg for at least 30 minutes, with a decreased cardiac index (CI) of 2.2 L/min or less, and a pulmonary artery occlusion pressure (PAOP) of 15 mm Hg or more.[2,5] When hemodynamic monitoring is unavailable, the diagnosis of cardiogenic shock can be made based on the clinical findings of hypotension or hypoperfusion as demonstrated by delayed capillary refill, decreased urinary output, and decreased level of consciousness, with cool and mottled extremities.[2]

CAUSES AND EPIDEMIOLOGY

Acute coronary syndrome (ACS) with myocardial infarction (MI) causing significant loss of myocardial functional ability, especially of the anterior wall of the left ventricle (LV), is the leading cause of cardiogenic shock.[2,6] Cardiogenic shock can also occur in patients with smaller infarctions, particularly if the person has suffered previous MIs. The cumulative effect of previous damage and new damage results in decreased pumping ability of the ventricle. Smaller infarctions with large areas of stunned or hibernating myocardium may also result in cardiogenic shock.[2]

Cardiogenic shock can result from a mechanical complication of AMI such as acute mitral valve regurgitation or rupture of the intraventricular septum. Other causes include isolated right ventricular (RV) failure, cardiac tamponade, cardiac rupture,

The author has nothing to disclose.

Baylor All Saints Medical Center, 1400 8th Avenue, Fort Worth, TX 76104, USA

E-mail address: Margaret.mcatee@baylorhealth.edu

Crit Care Nurs Clin N Am 23 (2011) 607–615

doi:10.1016/j.ccell.2011.09.001

Box 1
Causes of cardiogenic shock

- Acute myocardial infarction (most common)
- Mechanical complications of MI:
  - Acute mitral valve regurgitation
  - Rupture of the intraventricular septum
- Post-pump shock: myocardial depression after cardiopulmonary bypass
- Isolated RV failure
- Cardiac tamponade
- Cardiac rupture
- Myocarditis
- Acute decompensated heart failure
- End-stage cardiomyopathy
- Septic shock with myocardial depression
- Valvular heart disease
- Hypertrophic obstructive cardiomyopathy

Data from Josephson L. Cardiogenic shock. Dimens Crit Care Nurs 2008;27(4):160–70; and Tuggle D. Optimizing hemodynamics: strategies for fluid and medication titration in shock. In: Carlson KK, editor. AACN advanced critical care nursing. St. Louis (MO): Saunders Elsevier; 2009. p. 1099–133.

---

myocarditis, acute decompensated heart failure, end-stage cardiomyopathy, septic shock with severe myocardial depression, myocardial dysfunction after prolonged cardiopulmonary bypass, valvular heart disease, and hypertrophic obstructive cardiomyopathy.[2] Refer to **Box 1** for a list of the causes.

Characteristics of patients most likely to develop cardiogenic shock include older age, female sex, diabetic, anterior infarct, history of previous MI, peripheral vascular disease or prior cerebrovascular accident, decreased ejection fraction (EF), and larger MI as evidenced by higher cardiac enzyme levels.[2] There is also preliminary evidence that patients with a higher level of B-type natriuretic peptide (BNP) or its prohormone, Nt-pro BNP, within the first 24 hours of an ST elevation MI have a higher likelihood of developing cardiogenic shock, even if they are considered low risk according to other clinical parameters.[7]

PATHOPHYSIOLOGY

Development of cardiogenic shock is often directly related to the extent of damage to the myocardium. Autopsy studies demonstrate that in patients who lost at least 40% of LV muscle mass, cardiogenic shock resulted. In the setting of AMI, patients with an ST-elevation MI developed cardiogenic shock more frequently when compared to patients with a non-ST-elevation MI.[1] In cardiogenic shock, there is a syndrome of progressive deterioration because of a cycle of infarction resulting in a profound depression of cardiac output that causes further coronary insufficiency and loss of myocardial cells.[1]

An AMI causes myocardial cell death. When a critical mass of ventricular myocardial cells becomes ischemic or necrotic, the ventricle cannot pump effectively, leading

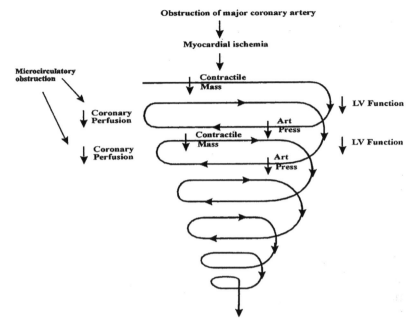

Fig. 1. The downward spiral of cardiogenic shock. (From Moscucci M, Bates ER. Cardiogenic shock. Cardiol Clin 1995;13(3):391–406; with permission.)

to a decrease in stroke volume and CO. With a decreased CO, diastolic blood pressure falls, causing a decrease in coronary perfusion pressure and decreased oxygen delivery to the myocardium. Hypotension ensues, which can cause a compensatory tachycardia to increase organ perfusion by attempting to increase CO. The tachycardia decreases diastolic filling time, thus further compromising blood flow to myocardial cells. Ischemia worsens, leading to a downward spiral that results in cardiogenic shock (**Fig. 1**).[2,8,9]

Decreased stroke volume means that the ventricle cannot eject a normal volume of blood with each contraction. Diastolic function of the ventricle is affected as well as the systolic function. The ventricular filling pressures and wall tension increase, resulting in increased myocardial oxygen demands. Increased filling pressures are reflected backward into the left atrium and pulmonary vessels, causing vascular congestion. If this continues, pulmonary edema occurs with impaired gas exchange.[2,9]

In the face of decreased CO and compromised tissue perfusion, compensatory mechanisms are activated. Sympathetic nervous system activation causes an increase in heart rate, as mentioned, as well as an increase in systemic vascular resistance (SVR) to improve CO and blood pressure. The renin–angiotensin–aldosterone system works to improve blood pressure by causing retention of sodium and water to increase intravascular volume. This causes an increase in preload. Although these compensatory mechanisms are helpful in shock states caused by hypovolemia, they are not helpful in cardiogenic shock and make the situation worse.[2,9]

Reversible Myocardial Dysfunction

There may be nonfunctioning areas of the heart that are still viable if appropriate treatment is initiated early. These areas with reversible dysfunction may have either hibernating or stunned myocardium.

Stunned myocardium consists of myocardial tissue that does not function normally after an ischemic event, even though normal perfusion to the area is restored. Normal function may return, but it takes time. Stunning may occur because of oxidative stress and interference with calcium homeostasis. There may also be a myocardial depressant factor that contributes to the situation. The degree of stunning is affected by the severity of the ischemia that occurred.[2]

Hibernating myocardium occurs because of a chronic decrease in coronary blood flow to an area. The body adapts by trying to balance the supply of oxygen with the demand. If normal blood flow is restored, the myocardial cells return to normal function.[2]

Changing Paradigm

In addition to the decreased contractile ability of the heart caused by ischemia and infarction, the development of cardiogenic shock is influenced by development of a systemic inflammatory response syndrome (SIRS) leading to the characteristic hemodynamic instability.[2,8,10] Twenty percent of patients in the SHOCK (**SH**ould we emergently revascularize **O**ccluded **C**oronaries in cardiogenic shoc**K**?) trial had signs and symptoms of SIRS, including fever and leukocytosis. Also, many of the patients did not have the expected increase in SVR. A low SVR was prognostic for an increased mortality.[2] The SHOCK trial demonstrated the importance of SIRS in the development of cardiogenic shock even in persons with only a modest decrease in EF.[1]

Almost one-half of nonsurvivors of cardiogenic shock die with a normal cardiac index (CI). This finding supports the paradigm of cardiogenic shock being more than just a cardiac problem but rather a disease of the entire circulatory system. The release of inflammatory mediators and neurohormones causes changes in the tissue microvasculature. These changes may result in multiorgan dysfunction syndrome (MODS) in cardiogenic shock.[3] SIRS also involves activation of complement, release of nitric oxide (NO), and release of inflammatory cytokines.[6] The NO leads to relaxation of smooth muscle and vasodilation. The vasodilation may be either beneficial or not. NO may combine with a substance called superoxide, a substance that forms during episodes of ischemia, to form peroxynitrate, a substance that is toxic to cells of the body. This combination may contribute to myocardial stunning and to continuation of the inflammatory process.[6]

TREATMENT

The long-term overall goal in managing cardiogenic shock is to decrease the myocardial workload to allow for cardiac recovery.[6] Because cardiogenic shock reflects a state of hypoperfusion induced by heart failure, management of cardiogenic shock should aim at optimizing tissue perfusion as well as improving cardiac function.[10] Because cardiogenic shock is usually a result of an AMI, early revascularization is recommended to interrupt the downward spiral of continued decrease in CO and hypoperfusion.[5,11]

Hemodynamic Monitoring

Intra-arterial pressure monitoring is recommended and pulmonary artery pressure (PAP) monitoring can be useful in managing patients with cardiogenic shock.[5] Calculating SVR can help determine if the patient is vasoconstricted or vasodilated so that appropriate treatment is implemented. The filling pressure that maintains the optimum CO is the goal.[2] Hemodynamic measurements such as PAOP and CO correlate with outcome, but

Table 1 CPO/CPI		
	Definition	**Formula**
CPO	The amount of energy available to maintain perfusion to vital organs in shock.	$CPO = MAP \times CO/451$
CPI	The amount of energy available to maintain perfusion to vital organs in shock indexed to body size.	$CPI = MAP \times CI/451$

are not associated with any benefit. There are various possible explanations for this. Some of the treatments currently used for patients with acute heart failure and cardiogenic shock were shown to improve symptoms but not final outcome. Titrating medications to achieve a set of predetermined hemodynamic goals might be actually detrimental to the patient. Perhaps the hemodynamic measures and their presumed target values used in treatment protocols are misleading.[12]

Forty-five percent (45%) of nonsurvivors of cardiogenic shock die with a normal cardiac index (ie, >2.2 L/min/m^2), indicating that improving macrohemodynamic parameters alone may not be enough to save the patient.[10] Cardiac power index (CPI) has been studied and may be a better marker of patient outcome.[3] Cardiac power (CPO) and CPI provide information about both cardiac function and tissue perfusion. CPO (**Table 1**) represents the amount of energy available to maintain perfusion to vital organs in shock.[3,12] CPO is calculated as $(MAP \times CO)/451$. CPI is calculated by substituting CI for CO: $CPI = (MAP \times CI)/451$.[12] By looking at the coupling of both pressure and flow of the cardiovascular system, CPO and CPI provide a measure of cardiac pumping.[12] A CPO less than or equal to 0.53 W and a CPI less than or equal to 0.8 W/m^2 have been shown to predict mortality.[12,13]

Circulatory Support: Drugs and Devices

Medications
Hypoperfusion may be treated initially with fluids to assess for hypovolemia unless the patient is in obvious pulmonary edema.[2] Use of a PA catheter may aid in fluid management. Inotropes and vasopressors are usually required to support blood pressure[2,5,6] American College of Cardiology/American Heart Association (ACC/AHA) guidelines recommend using dopamine 5 to 15 μg/kg/min IV for systolic blood pressure of 70 to 100 mm Hg with signs and symptoms of shock. If the systolic blood pressure is less than 70 mm Hg with signs and symptoms of shock, the guidelines recommend norepinephrine 0.5 to 30 μg/min. These two agents have both inotropic and vasopressor properties.[5]

Mechanical circulatory support
According to Abu-Omar, "The aim of [mechanical circulatory support] . . . in AMI complicated by cardiogenic shock is to restore cardiac output and preserve end-organ perfusion, off-load the ventricle, and optimize the balance between myocardial oxygen supply and demand, and allow for recovery of ischemic but viable myocardium."[1(p434)] Devices that may be used include an intra-aortic balloon pump (IABP), extracorporeal membrane oxygenation (ECMO), and ventricular assist devices (VAD). There are no large randomized control trials to validate their use in cardiogenic shock, but years of clinical experience indicate probable benefit.[1] It is important to remember that although these devices may help to stabilize a patient

in cardiogenic shock, revascularization is still necessary to restore optimum blood flow to affected myocardium.[2]

IABP

IABP is available in most centers in the United States. Inflation of the balloon in early diastole improves flow proximally to the coronary arteries and distally to the renal arteries. Deflation just before mechanical systole decreases afterload, thus decreasing LV workload and myocardial oxygen needs. Increased oxygen delivery to the myocardium improves contractility and CO. IABP is a Class 1 Level B recommendation for patients with an AMI who have cardiogenic shock that is not reversed by pharmacologic therapy.[5,6] One small single center study determined that insertion of the IABP before percutaneous coronary intervention (PCI) demonstrated improved morbidity and mortality compared to insertion after PCI. The benefit shown may be a result of improved coronary perfusion and unloading of the LV that may translate to significant salvaging of endangered myocardium.[14] Because treatment guidelines recommend door-to-balloon time of less than 90 minutes, IABP insertion is often delayed until the culprit vessel has been opened.[5,11]

Advantages of the IABP are its widespread availability and ease of insertion and management. Nursing care for patients receiving IABP therapy, in addition to the care required for the underlying situation, is focused on identification and prevention of device-related complications including bleeding, infection, ineffective augmentation, limb ischemia, and renal ischemia.[1,9]

Patients in cardiogenic shock who do not respond to pharmacologic and IABP therapy may benefit from more advanced circulatory support devices. Ideally, these devices should be implemented before end-organ failure occurs. Early implementation may prevent or reverse end-organ failure, minimize the size of the infarcted area, allow the myocardium to recover from the insult, and preserve myocardial function. One recommendation is that a mechanical circulatory device should be placed for patients who experience a continued low output state in the presence of two high-dose inotropic agents.[1] Patients with irreversible end-organ failure, including neurologic, are not candidates for these advanced devices. However, determining the critical timing of placement can be difficult.

ECMO

ECMO involves circulating the patient's blood through a circuit external to the body that includes a membrane oxygenator to reduce the contractile workload of the heart while maintaining adequate arterial oxygen content. ECMO provides support to both the RV and the LV. Cannulation of the femoral vein and artery can be performed at the bedside and can be done during cardiopulmonary resuscitation (CPR). For patients who have undergone coronary artery bypass graft (CABG) surgery, the cannulas can be placed centrally in the operating room while the chest is open. The advantages of ECMO over standard cardiopulmonary bypass are that it can be used for longer term support and the equipment is relatively easy to use and inexpensive. The effect on mortality is unclear. Some studies show improvement, while others do not. LV contractility should be maintained with inotropes to avoid ventricular stasis. Patients need to be anticoagulated during therapy to avoid thromboembolic events. Disadvantages of ECMO include lack of ready availability at all cardiac centers and complication risks that include limb ischemia, bleeding, infection, thromboembolism, and mechanical failure.[1,4,15,16]

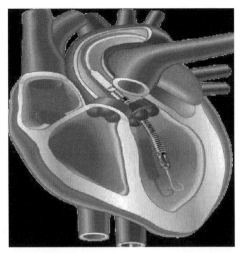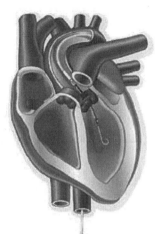

Fig. 2. Impella percutaneous LV assist device (Abiomed, Aachen, Germany). This device is inserted via a femoral artery and threaded up across the aortic valve. The inlet is located below the aortic valve and uses an axial pump that removes blood from the LV and ejects the blood via the outlet opening above the aortic valve. (*Courtesy of* Abiomed, Aachen, Germany.)

LVAD

An array of VADs are available. The choice depends on institutional device availability, operator experience, how urgently the patient requires support, the patient's general condition and treatment endpoints.[1] A VAD may be placed in either the LV, RV, or both depending on the patient needs. The advantage of a VAD over the IABP is full perfusion to the tissues to allow the heart to rest as opposed to an increase in CO of 10% to 20% with an IABP.[17] Patients who receive a LVAD early on may avoid the need for biventricular support, which has a poorer success rate. VADs may be implanted percutaneously or via sternotomy, depending on the model selected. One major disadvantage to VAD implantation is that they are not available at all centers. One study of a percutaneously inserted VAD demonstrated a complication rate that outweighed the benefit received from the VAD.[2] Complications include bleeding, disseminated intravascular clotting, infection including SIRS, and device failure.[2,17] The Impella (Abiomed, Aachen, Germany) percutaneous LVAD has been studied in patients with cardiogenic shock.[18] This device (**Fig. 2**) is placed via one of the femoral arteries and uses an axial pump that crosses the aortic valve. In the ISAR-SHOCK study, the Impella LP2.5 was compared to the IABP in patients with cardiogenic shock after an acute MI. Cardiac index was increased significantly after 30 minutes of support with the Impella LP2.5 compared with patients receiving IABP support. The Impella did not improve mortality but also did not cause increased bleeding or limb ischemia. The study may have been too small to demonstrate superiority of one device over another, but the fact that major complications and mortality were no different is reassuring.

Reperfusion therapy

In the presence of inadequate blood flow to the coronary arteries, inotropes alone will not improve hypotension. Coronary reperfusion strategies are the most effective treatment of cardiogenic shock.[2] Early revascularization has been shown to be superior to aggressive medical management and is recommended by the joint ACC/AHA guidelines.[1,5] Reperfusion can be done using PCI or CABG. PCI is available in many cardiac centers. In facilities without access to cardiac catheterization laboratories 24 hours a day, a system for rapid transfer of patients to a center with PCI availability should be in place. The advantage of PCI is the speed with which the coronary anatomy can be assessed and the culprit vessel opened. For patients with multivessel disease, the decision to intervene on other vessels may be delayed because of the patient's condition. Patients with lesions of the left main coronary artery may require CABG rather than PCI. CABG is also indicated for patients with multivessel disease or with acute mitral regurgitation associated with an MI. In this situation, the mitral valve should also be repaired.[2] Emergent surgical repair of other structural complications of AMI such as cardiac tamponade or septal defects should also be done.[6]

SUMMARY

Cardiogenic shock remains a significant issue and affects 5% to 10% of patients admitted with an AMI. Mortality remains high despite advances in treatment for AMI. These patients are best treated in centers where they can receive treatment that follows the joint guidelines recommended by ACC and AHA. Rapid reperfusion therapy as well as pharmacologic and mechanical circulatory support provide the best options for survival.

REFERENCES

1. Abu-Omar Y, Tsui SS. Mechanical circulatory support for AMI and cardiogenic shock. J Card Surg 2010;25:434–41.
2. Josephson L. Cardiogenic shock. Dimens Crit Care Nurs 2008;27(4):160–70.
3. Yilmaz MB, Mebazaa A. Searching for an ideal hemodynamic marker to predict short-term outcome in cardiogenic shock. Crit Care 2009;13(6):1013. Available at: http://ccforum.com/contenct/13/6/1013. Accessed January 16, 2011.
4. Liden H, Wiklund L, Haraldsson A, et al. Temporary circulatory support with extracorporeal membrane oxygenation in adults with refractory cardiogenic shock. Scand Cardiovasc J 2009;43:226–32.
5. Antman EM, Anbe DT, Armstrong PW, et al. ACC/AHA guidelines for the management of patients with ST-elevation myocardial infarction— executive summary: a report of the American College of Cardiology/American Heart Association task force on practice guidelines (writing committee to revise the 1999 guidelines for the management of patients with acute myocardial infarction). Circulation 2004;110;588–636. Available at: http://circ.ahajournals.org/cgi/content/full/110/5/588. Accessed January 21, 2011.
6. Tuggle D. Optimizing hemodynamics: strategies for fluid and medication titration in shock. In: Carlson KK, editor. AACN advanced critical care nursing. St. Louis (MO): Saunders Elsevier; 2009. p. 1099–133.
7. Jarai R, Huber K, Bogaerts K, et al. Prediction of cardiogenic shock using plasma B-type natriuretic peptide and the N-terminal fragment of its prohormone concentrations in ST elevation myocardial infarction: an analysis from the ASSENT-4 percutaneous intervention trial. Crit Care Med 2010;38(9)1793–801.
8. Prondzinsky R, Lemm H, Swyter M, et al. Intra-aortic balloon counterpulsation in patients with acute myocardial infarction complicated by cardiogenic shock: the prospective, randomized IABP SHOCK trial for attenuation of multiorgan dysfunction syndrome. Crit Care Med 2010;38(1)152–60.

9. Sice A. Intra-aortic balloon counterpulsation complicated by limb ischaemia: a reflective commentary. Nurs Crit Care 2006;11(6)297–304.
10. Den Uil CA, Lagrand WK, Valk S, et al. Management of cardiogenic shock: focus on tissue perfusion. Curr Probl Cardiol 2009;34:330–49.
11. Kushner FG, Hand M, Smith SC Jr, et al. 2009 focused updates: ACC/AHA guidelines for the management of patients with ST-elevation myocardial infarction (updating the 2004 guideline and 2007 focused update) and ACC/AHA/SCAI guidelines on percutaneous coronary intervention (updating the 2005 guideline and 2007 focused update): a report of the American College of Cardiology Foundation/American Heart Association task force on practice guidelines. J Am Coll Cardiol 2009;54:2205–41. Available at: http://content.onlinejacc.org/cgi/content/full/54/23/2205. Accessed September 8, 2011.
12. Fincke R, Hochman J, Lowe AM, et al. Cardiac power is the strongest hemodynamic correlate of mortality in cardiogenic shock: a report from the SHOCK trial registry. JACC 2004;44(2):340–8.
13. Torgersen C, Schmittinger CA, Wagner S, et al. Hemodynamic variables and mortality in cardiogenic shock: a retrospective cohort study. Crit Care 2009;13:R157.
14. Abdel-Wahab M, Saad M, Kynast J, et al. Comparison of hospital mortality with intra-aortic balloon counterpulsation insertion before versus after primary percutaneous coronary intervention for cardiogenic shock complicating acute myocardial infarction. Am J Cardiol 2010;105:967–71.
15. Rodriquez-Cruz E. Extracorporeal membrane oxygenation. Available at: http://emedicine.medscape.com. Accessed February 5, 2011.
16. Wu M, Lin P, Lee M, et al. Using extracorporeal support to resuscitate adult postcardiotomy cardiogenic shock: treatment strategies and predictors of short-term and midterm survival. Resuscitation 2010;81:1111–6.
17. Dirks JL. Cardiac surgery. In: Carlson KK, editor. AACN advanced critical care nursing. St. Louis (MO): Saunders Elsevier; 2009. p. 297–321.
18. Cove ME, MacLaren G. Clinical review: mechanical circulatory support for cardiogenic shock complicating acute myocardial infarction. Crit Care 2010;14:235–45.

Pulmonary Issues in Acute and Critical Care: Pulmonary Embolism and Ventilator-induced Lung Injury

Sonya Flanders, MSN, RN, ACNS-BC, CCRN[a,*],
Sharon Gunn, MSN, MA, RN, ACNS-BC, CCRN[b]

KEYWORDS

- Venous thromboembolism • Pulmonary embolism
- Nursing care • Ventilator-induced lung injury
- Ventilator-associated lung injury • Barotrauma
- Atelectrauma • Volutrauma • Biotrauma

PULMONARY EMBOLISM: CASE STUDY

TR, a 65-year-old obese white woman was admitted to the hospital one evening for progressive weakness and shortness of breath. TR's history included a remote non-ST elevation myocardial infarction and mild hypertension. On admission, she indicated she had not been taking her medications for the last several months and had spent the last week or more in bed or in her recliner. She was admitted to a telemetry unit for cardiac monitoring and observation because of a brief episode of chest pain in the emergency department after her initial electrocardiogram (ECG) and cardiac biomarkers were unremarkable, with a plan for continuous telemetry monitoring, serial laboratory values, and a cardiology consult in the morning. During the night, TR called out complaining of acute-onset chest pain and profound shortness of breath. Her blood pressure was 78/40 and decreasing, pulse 138, and respirations 36 breaths per minute. The nurse applied oxygen and called for emergency assistance. When the emergency team arrived, TR's blood pressure was 72/48, she remained severely short of breath and tachypneic, and her pulse oximeter reading was 68%.

The authors have nothing to disclose.

[a] Internal Medicine Services, Baylor University Medical Center, 3500 Gaston Avenue, Dallas, TX 75246, USA

[b] Critical Care Services, Baylor University Medical Center, 3500 Gaston Avenue, Dallas, TX 75246, USA

* Corresponding author.

E-mail address: sonya.flanders@baylorhealth.edu

The emergency team decided to intubate TR and transfer her to the intensive care unit for further interventions and stabilization.

BACKGROUND

Pulmonary embolism (PE) can be a serious and sometimes tragic event for patients across the health care continuum. PE occurs when an embolus obstructs one or more pulmonary arteries, which may result in partial or complete occlusion to distal pulmonary tissues.[1,2] The majority of PEs result from embolization of thrombi originating in the deep veins of the lower extremities or pelvis know as deep vein thrombosis (DVT), but some occur as a result of clots developing in arm veins or right cardiac chambers.[1] DVT and PE are manifestations of the overarching disease classification, venous thromboembolism (VTE). Aside from DVT, less-common sources of PE include fragments of tissue, amniotic fluid emboli, fat emboli, and air emboli.[2] This report focuses on PE arising from DVT.

VTE events are a significant health problem in the United States. In an epidemiologic review, White[3] reported approximately 100 first-time VTE events per 100 000 individuals in the United States annually. Altogether, it is estimated 900,000 VTE events occur each year.[4] Race appears to play a role in VTE, as Asian and Native Americans have a significantly lower risk for VTE events than white and black Americans.[4,5] Differences between sexes are less pronounced. Overall, men have a higher lifetime incidence rate of VTE than women, with a ratio of 1.2:1, although women have a slightly higher incidence than men during childbearing years.[4] VTE events increase exponentially with advancing age.[3] About two-thirds of VTE events involve only DVT, whereas one-third result in PE.[5]

Despite increasing awareness of VTE as a significant health concern, no significant changes in incidence of VTE have occurred for more than 2 decades.[4] Although advances in PE prevention strategies, diagnostics, and treatment modalities have occurred in recent years, 10% of patients die in the first 1 to 3 months after acute PE.[6] Sources indicate acute PE is the cause of death for 1% of patients admitted to hospitals, and 10% to 15% of all hospital deaths are related to PE.[1,6] Recently, The Joint Commission added VTE as one of the National Hospital Inpatient Quality Measures, which will likely serve to facilitate widespread implementation of assessment and prevention strategies in hospitals nationwide.[7] Acutely and critically ill patients often have 1 or more risk factors for VTE. Acute and critical care nurses need to be familiar with these risks as well as signs and symptoms, diagnostic tests, treatments, and, perhaps most importantly, prevention strategies for PE.

RISK FACTORS

Understanding the risks for VTE is essential nursing knowledge. Underlying etiology of VTE is linked to 3 physiologic components referred to as *Virchow's triad*: damage to the vascular endothelium, alterations in blood flow causing stasis, and hypercoagulability.[8]

A number of risk factors for the development of VTE have been identified, and some risks are more significant than others. Based on a review of 1231 patients requiring treatment for PE or acute DVT, the most frequent risk factor cited was age ≥ 40 years, accounting for 88.5% of this population.[8] In descending order, other risks identified in 10% or more of these subjects were obesity (37.8%), positive history for VTE (26%), cancer (22.3%), bed rest for 5 days or more (12%), and major surgery (11.2%).[8] Other risk factors included heart failure, varicose veins, hip or lower extremity fractures, estrogen therapy, stroke, multiple trauma, childbirth, and myocardial infarction.[8] The registered nurse who admitted TR identified several risk factors for VTE development. TR is obese, over the age of 40, and white. Additionally, she stated that she had spent the last week either in bed or in her recliner.

Anderson and Spencer[8] compiled VTE risk factors according to odds ratios; strong risk factors have an odds ratio greater than 10, moderate risk factors 2 to 9, and weak risk factors less than 2. Risk factors with the highest odds ratios include hip or lower extremity fracture, knee or hip replacement, major general surgery (eg, thoracic or abdominal surgeries utilizing general anesthesia for 30 minutes or longer), major trauma, and spinal cord injury.[8] Moderate risk factors are knee surgery via arthroscopy, central venous catheters, chemotherapy, heart or respiratory failure, hormone replacement therapy, malignancies, oral contraceptive use, paralytic stroke, pregnancy (postpartum), and thrombophilia.[8] The weakest risk factors are bed rest more than 3 days, immobility such as extended car or air travel, advancing age, laparoscopic surgical procedures, obesity, pregnancy (antepartum), and varicose veins.[8]

Numerous other risk factors have been reported in the literature. These include atrial fibrillation, acute myocardial infarction, nephrotic syndrome, acute infection, rheumatic disease, ischemic stroke, paraplegia, sickle cell anemia, inflammatory bowel disease, dehydration, systemic lupus erythematosus, inherited clotting disorders, family history of VTE, injection of substances that irritate endothelium, septic phlebitis, idiopathic thrombosis, and transvenous pacemakers.[1,2,4,9,10] Conversely, chronic liver disease reduces VTE risk.[4]

Although risk of VTE varies depending on predisposing patient characteristics and conditions, the cumulative effects of greater than 1 risk factor must also be taken into account. Hospitalization is an important risk factor for VTE events. It is valuable to note patients with surgical hospital admissions account for 24% of VTE events compared with 22% of VTE events occurring in patients hospitalized for medical reasons.[4] Health care team members must consider both populations when evaluating VTE risk.

Critical care nurses routinely encounter patients with preexisting VTE risk factors, but sometimes the risks increase due to care and treatments occurring in the intensive care unit (ICU), such as immobilization, paralytic medications, insertion of vascular access devices, dialysis, and sepsis.[11] Nurses play a crucial role in collaborating with other members of the health care team to offset VTE risks through assessment, and, when indicated, prophylaxis for VTE prevention.

PATHOPHYSIOLOGY

When one or more factors damages the vascular endothelium, alters blood flow leading to stasis, or results in hypercoagulability, a venous blood clot may form. PE occurs when the clot breaks free and lodges in the pulmonary circulation (**Figs. 1** and **2**). The physiologic response to this obstruction is an inflammatory response and release of several neurohumoral substances resulting in vasoconstriction.[2] Vasoconstriction serves to further reduce blood supply, compounding hypoperfusion to distal lung tissue and resulting in a ventilation-perfusion mismatch.[2] Although the affected tissue may be well ventilated, gas exchange is compromised because of decreased or absent circulation. Next, surfactant production decreases and leads to pulmonary edema and atelectasis, further exacerbating hypoxemia.[2] Pulmonary vascular resistance (PVR) increases, as does pulmonary artery pressure (PAP), which may lead to pulmonary hypertension and right-sided heart failure.[1]

PEs causing significantly reduced or absent blood flow to the lung tissue for long enough can lead to pulmonary tissue infarction.[2] After pulmonary infarction, scar tissue and atrophy of affected lung tissue leads to irreversible damage. Most

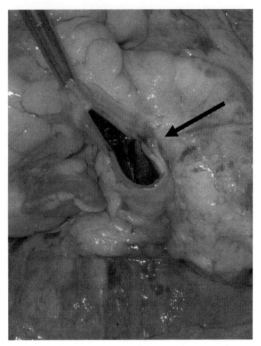

Fig. 1. The pulmonary trunk has been opened to reveal a large coiled thromboembolus extending from the heart toward the left lung. (*Courtesy of* Joseph M. Guileyardo, MD.)

less-significant PEs eventually dissolve without long-term impact on lung perfusion and function (**Fig. 3**).[2]

PREVENTION

The first step in nursing care for PE is avoidance, with a focus on DVT prevention. Several VTE prevention strategies can be used, including those aimed at advancing mobility, mechanical devices to reduce venous stasis risk, and pharmacologic interventions minimizing likelihood of clot formation. Nurses make a significant impact on prevention by planning care and implementing interventions to reduce VTE risks, such as facilitating early mobility by encouraging patients to ambulate and requesting consultations from physical medicine colleagues when appropriate. The value of mobility should not be overlooked and, in fact, for patients without VTE risk factors aside from minor general surgery procedures, early frequent ambulation is the only prophylaxis recommended.[11]

Because many patients are at risk for VTE, acute and critical care nurses should keep prevention top of mind. If there is no formal process for risk assessment and prophylaxis in place, nurses can champion creating policies, procedures, order sets, or other strategies in collaboration with physicians and pharmacists to ensure patients are screened for VTE risk and prophylaxis is initiated when appropriate.

Mechanical Prophylaxis

Mechanical prophylaxis techniques include graduated compression stockings, intermittent pneumatic compression devices, and foot pumps. Although evidence-based

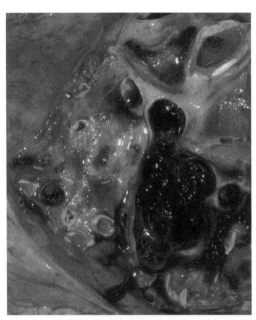

Fig. 2. A cross-section of the left lung hilum contains several large thromboemboli, which distend the vascular channels. (*Courtesy of* Joseph M. Guileyardo, MD.)

guidelines indicate mechanical prophylaxis has shown a reduction in DVT risk in certain populations, the effectiveness on PE and mortality risk is unknown, thus, mechanical devices should not be used in place of appropriate medications.[11] Mechanical prophylaxis in the absence of antithrombotic medications has a role for patients with moderate or high VTE risk and concomitant high risk of bleeding and may also be a useful adjunct to pharmacologic interventions for those with multiple VTE risk factors.[11]

Mechanical prophylactic devices must be used properly. For instance, nurses should ensure correct fit of stockings, taking leg measurements to select appropriate stocking size to optimize effectiveness. Mechanical devices vary and should be used according to manufacturer instructions. Some patients and families may be concerned about stockings making them feel hot or noise associated with mechanical devices. Patient and family education about the rationale for these treatments can help promote adherence.

Pharmacologic Prophylaxis

It makes sense that, because many hospitalized patients have risk factors for VTE, pharmacologic prophylaxis is recommended in patient populations with moderate to

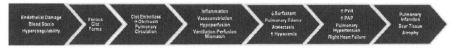

Fig. 3. An example of the pathophysiological sequence of pulmonary embolism.

Box 1
Selected categories of patient conditions with ACCP VTE prophylaxis recommendations[11]

- Acute spinal cord injury, trauma, burns
- Cancer
  - Undergoing surgery
  - Bedbound with acute medical illness
- Critically care admissions
- General Surgery
  - Bariatric
  - Coronary artery bypass
  - Gynecologic
  - Laparoscopic
  - Thoracic
  - Urologic
  - Vascular
- Medical conditions
  - Congestive heart failure
  - Severe respiratory disease
  - Other
- Neurosurgery
- Orthopedic procedures
  - Arthroscopic knee surgery
  - Elective hip replacement
  - Elective knee replacement
  - Elective spinal surgery
  - Hip fracture surgery

---

high VTE risk. These populations include those undergoing general surgery, orthopedic surgery, and neurosurgery; trauma patients; those with acute spinal cord injuries, medical conditions, or cancer; and patients admitted to critical care (**Box 1**).[11] Duration of treatment varies by population. When pharmacologic prophylaxis is indicated, patient-specific factors, including active bleeding, bleeding risk, age, and renal function need to be considered so risks and benefits of treatment can be weighed and adjustments made as necessary. For instance, in patients receiving neuraxial anesthesia or analgesia or deep peripheral nerve blocks, anticoagulant prophylaxis should be used with caution.[11] Detailed evidence-based guidelines for VTE prophylaxis based on patient risk stratification and surgical or medical conditions are published by the American College of Chest Physicians (ACCP) every few years.[11] Readers may wish to use this resource for more detailed information.

When indicated, appropriate medications for prophylaxis include either subcutaneous injections of low-dose unfractionated heparin (UFH), a low–molecular weight heparin (LMWH), or the pentasaccharide, fondaparinux, which inhibits factor X.[11]

Aspirin alone is not recommended.[11] Optimal medication choice and timing of initiation varies by population, so prophylaxis guidelines along with prescribing information should serve as references to clinicians. Patients should be screened for a history of adverse drug reactions, such as allergies and heparin-induced thrombocytopenia before initiation of prophylaxis, and positive screening results should be relayed to the prescriber. Once therapy has been initiated, nurses should assess patients for evidence of frank or occult bleeding and report signs of bleeding promptly. Hemoglobin level, hematocrit level, and platelet count should be monitored. Intramuscular injections and nonessential arterial and venous punctures are to be avoided. If spinal or epidural anesthesia or lumbar puncture is anticipated, the nurse should consult with the prescriber or proceduralist about holding anticoagulants before procedures.

Prophylactic doses of anticoagulants are generally lower than doses used for VTE treatment. For prophylaxis, 5000 units of subcutaneous UFH is administered 2 or 3 times daily.[9,12] A recent meta-analysis indicated UFH 3 times daily dosing was more effective in DVT prevention for hospitalized medical patients compared with twice-daily dosing.[13] LMWHs (eg, dalteparin, enoxaparin) and fondaparinux have the advantage of once-daily subcutaneous administration.[14,15] The standard enoxaparin dose is 30 mg or 40 mg once daily, depending on the type of surgical procedure or medical condition.[15] Prophylactic dosing of dalteparin also varies by indication, either 2500 or 5000 IU once daily.[14] LMWH dose adjustments are recommended for patients with impaired renal function and low body weight; liver function and age also should be considered.[12] If fondaparinux is prescribed for VTE prophylaxis, the dose is 2.5 mg once a day.[12] Fondaparinux is contraindicated when creatinine clearance is less than 30 mL/min.[9,12] Clinical pharmacists can be an invaluable resource to provide professional guidance when questions arise regarding dosing and monitoring of patients receiving anticoagulation.

RECOGNIZING SIGNS AND SYMPTOMS OF VTE

The majority of pulmonary emboli occur subsequent to embolization of DVT; however, DVT is typically asymptomatic.[2] Signs and symptoms associated with DVT include unilateral pain and swelling of the affected extremity, a palpable thrombus, or calf asymmetry of more than 1 cm.[2] Routine nursing assessments should include examinations for signs of VTE, and positive findings should be reported to the provider to facilitate prompt diagnostic testing and intervention.

Signs and symptoms of acute PE range from complete absence of symptoms to sudden death. The spectrum of presenting signs and symptoms may include tachycardia, tachypnea, shortness of breath, pleuritic-type chest pain, loud S_2 heart sound, audible S_3 and S_4, pulmonary wheezes or crackles, jugular venous distention, anxiety, and fever.[1,2] Signs and symptoms are related to the physiologic impact of the PE and depend on the degree of vascular obstruction, which pulmonary vessels are affected, and characteristics of the embolus.[2] For instance, complete obstruction of a main pulmonary artery carries significantly greater risk of deleterious effects to the patient than partial obstruction of a small distal pulmonary vessel because less lung tissue is affected. After PE, some patients go on to have chronic thromboembolic pulmonary hypertension and may exhibit signs of right heart failure: dyspnea on exertion, fatigue, and peripheral edema.[1]

Patients experiencing massive PE, such as TR, exhibit significant hypotension, tachycardia, pulmonary hypertension, chest pain, shock, and syncope.[1,2] These are ominous signs and often rapidly progress to cardiac arrest and death. As noted, sometimes PE is completely asymptomatic, but for nearly one-fourth of PE patients, death is the initial presentation, further highlighting the importance of prevention, early recognition, and swift interventions to improve patient outcomes.[5] Critical and acute care nurses know the signs and symptoms of massive PE are the same as some other cardiopulmonary emergencies, so rapid assessment of differential diagnoses must occur to guide treatment.

DIAGNOSIS OF PULMONARY EMBOLISM

If signs and symptoms of PE occur, diagnostic workup should occur swiftly. In acute care settings, readily available tests that may be part of the initial assessment include Spo_2 by pulse oximeter, arterial blood gases (ABG), 12-lead ECG, and chest x-ray.[1,2] Spo_2 and ABG are useful in detecting hypoxemia, and, if the patient is hyperventilating, the ABG result commonly shows respiratory alkalosis.[2] ECG findings may reveal right heart strain, tachycardia, nonspecific ST-T wave changes, right axis deviation, and inverted T-waves in leads V_1 through V_4.[1,2] Initial chest x-ray may be negative for abnormal findings or demonstrate nonspecific changes caused by atelectasis, pleural effusion, infiltrates, and elevated hemidiaphragm.[1]

Cardiac troponins may be elevated in PE as a result of right ventricular microinfarction, which has been associated with poor patient outcomes.[16] However, the value of troponins as a prognostic indicator may be limited: a recent meta-analysis led authors to conclude cardiac troponins are not helpful in stratifying risk of death in patients with normal blood pressures and acute symptomatic PE.[17]

Although none of these tests is specific to diagnose PE, all help provide further information about what may be transpiring in a symptomatic patient.

Several algorithms for diagnostic workup of PE are available to guide clinicians. The initial step is to determine clinical probability of PE based on risk assessment.[1,9,18] Clinical stability of the patient is also considered, because waiting for diagnostic screening tests could delay care for critically ill patients.

For patients at low risk and clinically stable, a D-dimer should be measured. A normal D-dimer precludes the need for further testing for PE, whereas an elevated result signals the need to proceed with imaging tests.[1,9,18] Clinically stable patients with high risk of PE should proceed directly to imaging studies.[9,19] This minimizes delays in care while awaiting D-dimer results. For hemodynamically unstable patients, rapid assessment with computed tomography (CT) is recommend if available; however, if not, or if the patient is too unstable for transport, bedside echocardiography to may be useful to visualize emboli in pulmonary arteries.[18]

Imaging options vary per institution. CT pulmonary angiogram is accurate and rapid, although because of the use of contrast, renal function and contrast allergies must be considered.[18,19] Ventilation-perfusion or V/Q lung scanning does not require contrast and is used to indentify lung tissue ventilated but not perfused, indicating V/Q mismatch. V/Q scans can be helpful by ruling out PE if results are entirely normal but are less useful in providing a firm positive diagnosis.[1,11] Pulmonary angiography is highly accurate but performed less frequently than in years past because of improvements in CT technology.

Another imaging test, duplex ultrasound scan, is not used to detect PE, rather, it examines extremities for DVT.[19] Limitations of duplex ultrasound scan are that accuracy varies by operator, DVT in the pelvis or calf veins cannot be detected realibily, and edema and obesity impede accuracy.[9] A positive ultrasound scan means anticoagulation is indicated, whereas a negative ultrasound scan indicates further workup should occur.[1]

TREATMENT OF PULMONARY EMBOLISM

Initial treatment of acute PE should be tailored per patient based on physiologic condition. Basic actions are administration of oxygen and ensuring the patient has a patent intravenous (IV) line. Patients with significant cardiorespiratory compromise and shock need advanced life support such as vasopressors, endotracheal intubation, and mechanical ventilation. For hemodynamically unstable patients, nurses should prepare to rapidly administer medications and transport patients to procedure areas or a higher level of care. Swift dissolution of clot is crucial in the setting of PE with hemodynamic instability, which carries a 58% rate of death versus 15% in hemodynamically stable patients.[18] Patients who have right ventricular failure leading to refractory hypotension have higher mortality than those who do not. [6] Prompt treatment of hemodynamically compromised patients has been shown to reduce mortality risk to less than 30%.[18]

Specific, evidence-based recommendations for treatment of VTE are in the ACCP guidelines and should be consulted for those wishing more detailed information.[16] An overview of treatment options for acute PE follows.

Anticoagulation

Treatment with anticoagulation should commence upon diagnosis of acute PE and in cases with high suspicion of PE while waiting for diagnostic confirmation.[16] Anticoagulants act to prevent further clot formation and extension of existing clots. Anticoagulants recommended in ACCP evidence-based guidelines for treatment of VTE include therapeutic dosing with subcutaneous fixed-dose or monitored UFH, intravenous UFH, or subcutaneous LMWH or fondaparinux.[16] Therapeutic doses of anticoagulants generally are higher than those used for prophylaxis. Nursing implications and monitoring considerations are the same as those discussed for prophylaxis.

IV heparin is the preferred anticoagulant for massive PE or when thrombolysis is being planned or considered, with an initial IV bolus of 80 units/kilogram (kg) or 5000 units followed immediately by continuous IV heparin starting at 18 units/kg per hour or 1300 units per hour. Laboratory monitoring of activated partial thromboplastin time or heparin assay is necessary to guide dose adjustments to achieve desired therapeutic response.

Tinzaparin is a factor X inhibitor not discussed previously in this report, as it is not labeled for VTE prophylaxis but is indicated for acute DVT treatment with or without PE.[9,12] Tinzaparin should be used with caution for elderly patients, in diabetic retinopathy, and in the setting of renal insufficiency.[20] The once-daily subcutaneous dose of tinzaparin is 175 anti-Xa international units per kilogram.[9,20]

Initiating a vitamin K antagonist (VKA), such as warfarin, along with parenteral anticoagulation is recommended with concurrent therapy for 5 days minimum until international normalized ratio (INR) is 2.0 or greater for at least 24 hours.[16] Practically speaking, early warfarin initiation may be limited in critically ill patients because of inability to take oral medications. Newer oral anticoagulants may eventually have a role in VTE standards.[21] At this time, none of these agents is approved for VTE prevention or treatment in the United States, but nurses should be aware that new medication options may emerge.

Thrombolysis

Unlike anticoagulants, thrombolytic agents actively degrade existing clots by converting plasminogen to plasmin. Thrombolytics are not indicated for all patients with PE, but should be considered in the setting of acute PE.[16] Recent publications suggest thrombolytics are useful in hemodynamically unstable patients (ie, hypotension with systolic blood pressure [SBP] <90 mm Hg or decline in SBP by >40 mm Hg from baseline lasting 15 minutes or more, and decreased end-organ perfusion) or if vasopressors are required to maintain SBP of 90 mm Hg or greater.[6,18] Agnelli and Becattini[18] suggest thrombolytic treatment in acute PE with hypotension when patients are hemodynamically stable but have clear signs of RV failure by echocardiography. ACCP guidelines advocate for thrombolytics in high-risk PE without hypotension as long as bleeding risk is low.[16] Further studies on thrombolytic use are recommended to guide risks and benefits in hemodynamically stable patients, and current guidelines suggest the majority of patients with PE should not receive thrombolytics.[16]

In hemodynamically unstable patients, delays in thrombolytics may lead to irreversible organ damage caused by hypoperfusion, thus, timeliness is critical.[16] When thrombolytics are indicated, they are used in conjunction with anticoagulants and should be administered as early as possible after PE diagnosis.[6] Some analyses indicate thrombolytic use is associated with a reduction in mortality and an increased risk of major bleeding.[16] Risks and benefits always must be evaluated as part of patient selection. Because of risk for bleeding, patients need to be screened for absolute and relative contraindications before administration. Absolute contraindications are intracranial hemorrhage (current or historical), neoplasm, aneurysm or arteriovenous malformation; major head trauma; bleeding disorder; and active internal bleeding within 3 months of intracranial or intraspinal surgery and within 2 months of cerebrovascular accident.[22] Relative contraindications are recent internal bleeding, organ biopsy, surgery, or trauma including cardiopulmonary resuscitation; venipuncture via a noncompressible location; uncontrolled hypertension; high risk of left cardiac thrombosis; pregnancy; diabetic retinopathy; and age older than 75 years.[22] Nurses administering thrombolytics should be familiar with contraindications and may participate in screening alongside other health care team members to facilitate rapid initiation of the prescribed medication. A thrombolytic screening checklist is one strategy to consider in expediting complete assessment for contraindications.

Recombinant tissue plasminogen activator, 100 mg over 2 hours via peripheral IV, has been studied and used more than other thrombolytic regimens and has been associated with less bleeding than longer infusion times of 12 or 24 hours and direct infusions into the pulmonary artery.[16] During infusion, IV UFH may be held temporarily but should be restarted once thrombolytic administration is complete.[16]

Other thrombolytic agents and regimens have been studied, but availability and approved indications vary. Thrombolytic selection may depend on the prescriber and facility, for instance, because of hospital medication formularies. Nurses need to know that dosing of thrombolytic agents differs by agent and indication. PE order sets outlining standardized regimens for thrombolytic administration can help facilitate dosing accuracy and minimize delays in care.

Vena Cava Filter

A filter may be placed in the vena cava to trap any emboli in patients with contraindications to anticoagulation or in those who have DVT or PE despite anticoagulation.[19] Most filters are placed in the inferior vena cava (IVC); however, if the origin of thrombus is an upper extremity, a filter may be placed in the superior vena cava.[19] Risks and benefits of IVC filters are unclear, and insertion has been associated with increased VTE risk over time; therefore, current guidelines discourage routine IVC placement unless anticoagulation is contraindicated because of bleeding risk, and recommend ongoing patient re-evaluation for anticoagulation if bleeding risk resolves.[16]

Catheter-based Thrombus Removal

Catheter-based thrombus removal involves use of a catheter to break up or remove the thrombus. Different catheters and techniques are available, including clot fragmentation, pulverization, and extraction. Availability of these catheter-based interventions varies by facility depending on access to necessary equipment and qualified proceduralists. Research to support use of these techniques is limited, but available literature suggests lives have been saved following catheter-based interventions in the setting of massive PE; therefore, ACCP guidelines recommend these techniques be reserved for severely compromised patients who have contraindications to or cannot tolerate delays associated with thrombolysis if experts are available.[16]

Surgical Interventions

Pulmonary surgical embolectomy involves surgical removal of a thrombus in the operating room using cardiopulmonary bypass.[16] In some cases, rescue surgery may be attempted if thrombolysis fails. Guidelines for surgical embolectomy mirror those for catheter-based interventions: severely compromised patients with contraindications to or inability to tolerate delays associated with thrombolysis when expert surgeons are available.[16] A recent report of favorable mortality outcomes after aggressive surgical pulmonary embolectomy in 18 high-risk patients led authors to suggest earlier surgical intervention in the setting of right ventricular dysfunction before progression to severe hemodynamic compromise may improve outcomes.[23]

Long-term Treatment

After PE, patients should expect to continue anticoagulation for at least 3 months, depending on circumstances.[16] If a reversible risk factor provoked PE and has been corrected, 3 months of therapy with a VKA (eg, warfarin) is recommended, but if VTE was unprovoked, a risk-benefit analysis for long-term therapy is advised. When risk of bleeding is low, long-term treatment is preferred, with re-evaluation as part of ongoing follow-up care. Recommendations for patients with cancer and PE differ from those without cancer: LMWH therapy is recommended for at least 3 to 6 months, followed by conversion to a VKA or continuation of LMWH long-term or until resolution of cancer.[16] Patients taking warfarin need periodic laboratory testing to monitor INR with a target therapeutic INR range of 2.0 to 3.0.[16] When patients are started on long-term anticoagulation, nursing interventions include providing patient and family education. The Joint Commission Core Measures for VTE and 2011 National Patient Safety Goal 03.05.01 specify patient education about warfarin must include compliance issues, dietary advice, need for follow-up monitoring, and adverse drug reactions and drug interactions.[24,25] Nurses should become familiar with regulatory expectations, provide patients and families with effective education before hospital discharge, evaluate comprehension, and document education provided in the medical record.

CASE STUDY

Upon transfer to the ICU, TR is started on therapeutic IV heparin. She requires norepinephrine to maintain her SBP above 90 mm Hg. A portable chest x-ray confirmed correct placement of her endotracheal tube and found signs of pulmonary edema. TR is transported emergently for a CT pulmonary angiogram, which confirms a large PE. Upon return to the ICU TR is placed on a volume-controlled mode of

---

Box 2
Ventilator induced lung injury terminology[48]

- Barotrauma—alveolar damage caused by increased pressures in the lung
- Volutrauma—alveolar damage caused by increased volumes in the lung
- Atelectrauma—damage to lung caused by repeated alveolar collapse (derecruitment) and inflation (recruitment)
- Biotrauma—release of chemical mediators caused by alveolar damage

---

ventilation. The receiving nurse initiates a propofol drip titrated to keep TR minimally sedated. An initial assessment is performed, and lung sounds are slightly diminished with minimal crackles. TR has no contraindications for thrombolytic therapy, so infusion of tissue plasminogen activator is initiated promptly, during which heparin is temporarily suspended. Vital signs are recorded and ventilator settings are verified. TR denies shortness of breath, chest pain, and anxiety. Nursing priorities include implementation of current evidence-based practices to maintain patient safety and prevent any iatrogenic complications. The ventilator bundle is initiated to minimize the patient's risk of acquiring ventilator-associated pneumonia. Nursing measures include elevation of the head of the bed, routinely scheduled oral care, daily sedation vacations, and assessment of weaning readiness.[26]

THE BASICS OF MECHANICAL VENTILATION

The pulmonary system delivers oxygen into the bloodstream for distribution throughout the body. This is accomplished in 2 ways: ventilation, and diffusion of oxygen across an alveolar membrane into the bloodstream. Respiratory failure occurs when the patient cannot get air into or out of the lungs or when air that gets into the lungs cannot diffuse into the bloodstream.

Patients are placed on mechanical ventilation to facilitate oxygenation in pathologic respiratory states, for airway support during operative procedures, and airway protection due to other disease processes when the patient may not be able to protect their airway. Inspiratory breaths are delivered by forcing air into the lungs at predetermined volumes or pressures, hence the term *positive pressure ventilation*. Exhalation is a passive process, similar to spontaneous breathing.[27]

RISKS OF MECHANICAL VENTILATION

Mechanical ventilation can be a life-saving intervention and is sometimes necessary for airway protection, but it is not without potential problems. Patients intubated for operative procedures or airway protection may not have underlying respiratory disease but are still at risk for complications of mechanical ventilation. Add an already injured lung into the mix and care becomes even more complex. Complications of positive pressure mechanical ventilation are known as ventilator-induced lung injury (VILI). There are 4 causes of VILI: barotrauma, volutrauma, atelectrauma, and biotrauma (**Box 2**). VILI can lead to acute lung injury (ALI), adult respiratory distress syndrome (ARDS), multisystem organ failure, and death.[28] Acute lung injury caused by inappropriate ventilator settings is a common cause of respiratory failure and has a high mortality rate, exceeding 45% in some studies.[29,30]

Lung injury associated with inappropriate or suboptimal ventilator settings is not always at the forefront of the clinician's mind during routine daily nursing care, especially when the focus is on managing patient illness. Awareness and understanding of the risks of mechanical ventilation are the first steps in providing safe care and are valuable components of proactive and competent professional nursing practice.

Ventilator settings or modes of mechanical ventilation are determined based on patient need, patient tolerance, and physician practice. In general, there are 2 modes: controlled and assisted. In controlled modes, the ventilator initiates the breath and takes over all the work of breathing. In assisted modes the patient may initiate a breath, and the ventilator provides varying support for work of breathing. Additionally, breaths may be delivered via volume or pressure settings. Simply put, volume modes deliver a preset tidal volume to the patient each breath, whereas pressure modes are based on the compliance and airway resistance in the patient's lungs. Lung compliance basically refers to the elasticity of the lungs. Healthy lungs are more compliant and distensible. Diseased or damaged lungs become less compliant or "stiff." This can become challenging when trying to ventilate a patient with very stiff lungs, such as in the setting of ARDS. Airway resistance increases with airway constriction or blockage. The higher the airway resistance, the more difficult it is to ventilate. Problems in ventilation may be getting oxygen into the lungs, getting carbon dioxide out, or both.

In volume modes, the tidal volume remains constant with each breath, but pressures within the lung vary. The patient with stiffer, less compliant lungs will require more pressure to ventilate a 500-mL tidal volume than a patient with more elastic lungs.

Conversely, in pressure modes, a predetermined maximum pressure setting on inspiration prevents lung damage caused by excessive pressure, but lung volumes vary with each breath. Modern ventilation strategies have evolved so volume and pressure modes may be combined and tailored to the individual patient needs and tolerances.[31,32] Manipulating ventilator settings to individual patient needs are important in preventing VILI.

There are some common terminologies that are necessary to define to facilitate a deeper understanding of mechanical ventilation and patient care. Positive end-expiratory pressure (PEEP) is used to increase the amount of air remaining in a patient's lungs at end expiration. This remaining air keeps more alveoli open for gas exchange and decreases any effort the patient may have to make to reopen alveoli that collapse at end expiration; however, PEEP may also cause increased intrathoracic pressure, decreased cardiac output, increased air trapping, and risk of volutrauma.[33]

Inspiratory-to-expiratory ratio (I:E ratio) is the amount of time allocated to inspiration and expiration with each breath.[33] During normal breathing, the I:E ratio is 1:2. With mechanical ventilation, these ratios can be manipulated to support patient needs. For example, if the patient is retaining carbon dioxide (CO_2) the ratio could be changed to 1:3, allowing more time for exhalation to help decrease CO_2 levels. Altering the I:E ratio may require the patient receive more sedation, as this goes against the instinctual breathing pattern.

Tidal volume is the amount of gas delivered in 1 breath. This is usually calculated based on a patient's ideal body weight. Over the last 2 decades, practice guidelines have emerged supporting lower tidal volumes. This will be explained in greater detail in later discussion. Let us now take a closer look at complications associated with mechanical ventilation.

CASE STUDY

Six hours after completion of the thrombolytic, TR's blood pressure and heart rate have stabilized allowing the norepinephrine to be weaned off, The critical care nurse notes that TR's oxygen saturation levels are dropping. TR also is becoming more anxious and agitated. Suspecting the patient needs suctioning, the nurse auscultates TR's lungs bilaterally and notes increased crackles. Suctioning does not resolve the issue, so the nurse notifies the physician who orders a chest x-ray and ABG. X-ray results reveal increased pulmonary infiltrates and a worsening hypoxemia. Collaboratively, the nurse and physician suspect that volutrauma may be worsening the patient's pulmonary condition. The physician decreases the patient's tidal volume, increases the respiratory rate, and adjusts PEEP settings to 10 cm H_2O.

Volutrauma

Patients placed on volume modes of mechanical ventilation are at risk of volutrauma. Volutrauma is overdistension of the alveoli due to too much volume being delivered. Alveoli in the lungs are not uniformly inflated. Atelectasis and disease states can leave some areas of lung nonventilated. As a result, the volume delivered is then dispersed to the healthy areas of the lung causing the overdistension of healthy alveoli. Overstretching of the alveoli causes damage at the cellular level, initiating the inflammatory response and increasing cellular permeability.[34] Clinically, the patient presents with a noncardiogenic pulmonary edema.[35]

Ventilation of patients using lower tidal volumes was highlighted in a landmark study conducted by ARDS network in the late 1990s.[36] This study compared the impact of traditional tidal volumes of 12 mL/kg versus smaller tidal volumes of 6 mL/kg in the outcomes of patients with ARDS. The mortality outcomes of patients receiving lower tidal volumes were so much better than the comparison group that the study was stopped early. Since that time, lower tidal volumes have become standardized practice in clinical settings.[28,29,37,38]

CASE STUDY

As night shift approaches, the nurse notes TR's peak airway pressures trending upward. The patient is anxious and has increased work of breathing. The nurse knows TR is at risk for complications of barotrauma, and collaborates with the physician as she makes her last rounds for the day. The physician switches to a bi-level pressure mode on the ventilator. The patient seems to tolerate this mode and relaxes. Oxygen saturation levels increase, and the nurse records tidal volumes with hourly vital signs.

Barotrauma

Positive pressure ventilation can result in barotrauma because of high airway pressures in the lung.[34] These high pressures may be caused by excessive levels of PEEP or high inspiratory pressures.[39] Barotrauma will develop in up to 20% of mechanically ventilated patients with an associated mortality risk of 70% to 80%.[40] High pressures in the lung cause the alveoli to overdistend, which occasionally leads to alveolar rupture. The result is a pneumothorax, tension pneumothorax, pneumomediastinum, subcutaneous emphysema, or other types of air-leaking into the patient's tissues.[28,40] The patient may present clinically with dyspnea, chest pain, or decreased breath sounds on 1 side of the chest. Puffy tissue, which reveals crepitus on palpation, may be indicative of subcutaneous emphysema. If crackles occur in rhythm with the pulse and are not associated with the respiratory cycle, pneumomediastinum should be suspected, which is a medical emergency. The astute nurse will monitor ventilator volumes and pressures on an ongoing basis and regularly assess the patient for potential complications. If airway pressures are trending upward or if the patient is becoming restless, an attempt should be made to identify the cause.

The daily chest x-ray is often the earliest indication that barotrauma has occurred. An increased risk of barotrauma development has also been linked to higher tidal volumes.[41]

CASE STUDY

The ICU nurse leaves for the evening and comes back to her assignment the following morning. Overnight TR's condition has worsened. The morning chest x-ray shows increased bilateral infiltrates and atelectasis. Blood gas results show worsening hypoxemia. The patient is now heavily sedated on a reverse I:E ratio. The prolonged inspiratory time allows the ventilator to deliver oxygen at a preset pressure limit over a longer period of time. The nurse knows that VILI may be the culprit for TR's deterioration.

Atelectrauma

Atelectasis is the partial or complete collapse of alveoli in the lungs, which compromises airflow and gas exchange at the cellular level. Atelectasis has numerous causes, including mechanical ventilation, mucous plugging, pulmonary embolus, and injury to the lung from disease or trauma.[42]

When alveoli collapse at the end of expiration, increased force is needed to reopen them for the next inspiratory breath. This collapsing and reopening causes injury to the lung through shearing and is known as *atelectrauma*.[34] Reopening of the collapsed alveoli is commonly referred to as *recruitment* of the lung and may be a more familiar terminology to the clinician.[39] Ironically, low tidal volumes can result in alveolar collapse. So here we have one of those conundrums in health care: lower the tidal volume to prevent volutrauma at the risk of causing atelectrauma! Clinical solutions to avoid large tidal volumes while minimizing atelectrauma are to add PEEP to the ventilator settings or to prolong inspiratory time in pressure mode ventilation. PEEP helps to keep the alveoli open at end exhalation, and prolonging peak inspiratory pressure holds the alveoli open and promotes recruitment of additional alveolar sacs.[43] Fortunately, current ventilator technologies offer many modes that can be tailored to individual patient needs.[44] From a nursing perspective, prevention and early recognition is key. Physical assessment findings in the patient with atelectasis may include tachycardia, decreased breath sounds, crackles, or dyspnea. Diagnostic tests such as ABGs and chest x-rays may be ordered to reinforce these findings. Frequent turning, auscultation of breath sounds, and suctioning to remove mobilized secretions are fundamental nursing interventions. It is important to minimize or eliminate any breaks in the ventilator circuit, as even 1 breath without PEEP can cause alveolar collapse.[34] Routine tracheal saline installation should also be avoided, as this worsens derecruitment and increases pressures needed to reopen collapsed alveoli.[43]

Biotrauma

Biotrauma is the release of chemical mediators caused by overstretching, shearing, or excessive inspiratory pressures during mechanical ventilation. These chemical mediators cause both pulmonary and systemic inflammation.[45,46] Damage to the endothelial cells in the alveoli results in increased permeability translocation of bacteria into the systemic circulation and multiorgan system failure in severe cases.[34,39,47] Research in this particular area is in its infancy. Identification of specific biological and inflammatory markers may help clinicians intervene earlier to prevent systemic organ damage.[46] Important nursing considerations are observing for signs and symptoms of systemic inflammatory response syndrome (SIRS) and monitoring organ function distal to the lungs.

CASE STUDY

For the remainder of the shift, TR's nurse insures nursing interventions focus on delivering safe patient care. Infection prevention strategies and routine turning to promote alveolar recruitment are priorities. Routine assessments and monitoring of TR's response to therapy facilitate a proactive approach to care.

On TR's second day in the ICU, a bedside transesophageal echocardiogram is performed to evaluate the status of her PE. Images show complete dissolution of the clot. Intravenous heparin is continued.

Over the next few days, ventilator settings continue to be adapted as her condition changes. The exemplary care provided by the health care team pays off. On day 7 of ventilator support, TR is extubated. She is transferred back to a telemetry unit the following day for continuous cardiac monitoring, when IV heparin is discontinued and she is started on a LMWH and warfarin. The Physical Therapy Department is consulted to aid with mobility and physical conditioning.

TR improves significantly over the next several days and is discharged home with her husband. The discharging nurse ensures both TR and her husband are clear on instructions to follow up with her primary care provider for anticoagulation monitoring and understand key self-care concepts related to warfarin therapy. The nurse also verifies outpatient physical therapy is arranged as ordered by the physician. TR and her husband express gratitude for the care she has received from the entire care team in the hospital, including the exceptional care of her acute and critical care nurses.

SUMMARY

Many patients admitted to acute care hospitals are at risk for VTE. Nurses play a pivotal role in prevention of VTE events by assessing risk and implementing prophylactic interventions, promptly recognizing and reacting to signs and symptoms of DVT and PE, and collaborating with other team members to ensure rapid treatment ensues. When patients require mechanical ventilation, nurses need to remain alert for complications indicative of VILI, effectively communicate assessment findings to other team members and confidently implement nursing and ordered medical interventions to promote the best possible patient outcomes.

REFERENCES

1. Beers MH, Porter RS, Jones T, et al, editors. The Merck manual of diagnosis and therapy. 18th edition. Whitehouse Station (NJ): Merck Research Laboratories; 2006.
2. Brashers VL. Alterations of pulmonary function. In: McCance KLH, Huether SE, editors. Pathophysiology: the biologic basis for disease in adults and children. 5th edition. Philadelphia: Elsevier Mosby; 2006.
3. White RH. The epidemiology of venous thromboembolism. Circulation 2003;107:I4–8.
4. Heit JA. The epidemiology of venous thromboembolism in the community. Arterioscler Thromb Vac Biol 2008;28:370–2.
5. White RH, Zhou H, Romano PS. Incidence of symptomatic venous thromboembolism after different elective or urgent surgical procedures. Thromb Haemost 2003;90:446–55.

6. Lankeit M, Konstantinides S. Mortality risk assessment and the role of thrombolysis in pulmonary embolism. Clin Chest Med 2010;31:759–69.

7. The Joint Commission. Venouos thromboembolism.2009. Available at: http://www. jointcommission.org/venous_thromboembolism/. Accessed January 15, 2011.

8. Anderson F Jr, Spencer F. Risk factors for venous thromboembolism. Circulation 2003;107:I9–16.

9. Dirks JL, Howland-Gradman J. Vascular emergencies. In: Carlson KK, editor. AACN advanced critical care. St. Louis: Saunders Elsevier; 2009. p. 347–83.

10. Alikhan R, Spyropoulos AC. Epidemiology of venous thromboembolism in cardiorespiratory and infectious disease. Am J Med 2008;121:935–42.

11. Geerts WH, Bergqvist D, Pineo GF, et al. Prevention of venous thromboembolism: American College of Chest Physicians evidence-based clinical practice guidelines. 8th edition. Chest 2008;133:381S–453S.

12. Deglin JH, Vallerand AH. Fondaparinux. Philadelphia: F.A. Davis Company; 2011.

13. Wein L, Wein S, Haas SJ, et al. Pharmacological venous thromboembolism prophylaxis in hospitalized medical patients: a meta-analysis of randomized controlled trials. Arch Intern Med 2007;167:1476–86.

14. Deglin JH, Vallerand AH. Dalteparin. Philadelphia: F.A. Davis Company; 2011.

15. Deglin JH, Vallerand AH. Enoxaparin. Philadelphia: F.A. Davis Company; 2011.

16. Kearon C, Kahn S, Agnelli G, et al. Antithrombotic therapy for venous thromboembolic disease. Chest 2008;133:454S–545S.

17. Jiménez D, Uresandi F, Otero R, et al. Troponin-based risk stratification of patients with acute nonmassive pulmonary embolism: systematic review and metaanalysis. Chest 2009;136:974–82.

18. Agnelli G, Becattini C. Acute pulmonary embolism. N Engl J Med 2010;363:266–74.

19. Yang JC. Prevention and treatment of deep vein thrombosis and pulmonary embolism in critically ill patients. Crit Care Nurs Q 2005;28:72–9.

20. Deglin JH, Vallerand AH. Tinzaparin. Philadelphia: F.A. Davis Company; 2011.

21. Merli GJ. New oral antithrombotic agents for the prevention of deep venous thrombosis and pulmonary embolism in orthopedic surgery. Orthopedics 2010;33:27S–32S.

22. Todd JL, Tapson VF. Thrombolytic therapy for acute pulmonary embolism. Chest 2009;135:1321–9.

23. Sareyyupoglu B, Greason KL, Suri RM, et al. A more aggressive approach to emergency embolectomy for acute pulmonary embolism. Mayo Clin Proc 2010;85: 785–90.

24. The Joint Commission. Accreditation manual: hospital. National patient safety goals. 2011. Available at: http://www.jointcommission.org/assets/1/6/2011_NPSGs_HAP. pdf. Accessed January 21, 2011.

25. The Joint Commission. Specifications manual for national hospital inpatient quality measures. October 20, 2010; Version 3.2:VTE-5-1 - VTE 5-6. Available at: http://www.jointcommission.org/specifications_manual_for_national_hospital_inpatient_ quality_measures/. Accessed January 21, 2011.

26. Grap MJ. Not-so-trivial pursuit: mechanical ventilation risk reduction. Am J Crit Care 2009;18:299–309.

27. Pierce LNB. Invasive and noninvasive modes and methods of mechanical ventilation. In: Burns S, editor. AACN protocols for practice: care of mechanically ventilated patients. 2nd edition. Sudbury (MA): Jones and Bartlett; 2007. p. 59–94.

28. Donahoe M. Basic ventilator management: lung protective strategies. Surg Clin North Am 2006;86:1389–408.

29. Gajic O, Dara SI, Mendez JL, et al. Ventilator-associated lung injury in patients without acute lung injury at the onset of mechanical ventilation. Crit Care Med 2004;32:1817–24.

30. Fernández-Pérez ER, Sprung J, Afessa B, et al. Intraoperative ventilator settings and acute lung injury after elective surgery: a nested case control study. Thorax 2009;64: 121–7.

31. Pertab D. Principles of mechanical ventilation—a critical review. Br J Nurs 2009;18: 915–8.

32. Fenstermacher D. Hong D. Mechanical ventilation: what have we learned? Crit Care Nurs Q 2004;27:258–94.

33. Newmarch C. Caring for the mechanically ventilated patient: part one. Nurs Stand 2006;20:55.

34. Pinhu L, Whitehead T, Evans T, et al. Ventilator-associated lung injury. Lancet 2003;361:332–40.

35. Schultz MJ, Haitsma JJ, Slutsky AS, et al. What tidal volumes should be used in patients without acute lung injury? Anesthesiology 2007;106:1226–31.

36. ARDSNet. ARMA Study. 2000. Available at: http://www.ardsnet.org/studies/arma. Accessed January 10, 2011.

37. Bigatello LM, Pesenti A. Ventilator-induced lung injury: less ventilation, less injury. Anesthesiology 2009;111:699–700.

38. Mackay A, Al-Haddad M. Acute lung injury and acute respiratory distress syndrome. Continuing Education in Anaesthesia, Critical Care & Pain 2009;9:152–6.

39. Cooper SJ. Methods to prevent ventilator-associated lung injury: a summary. Int Crit Care Nurs 2004;20:358–65.

40. Schub T, Buckley BL. Barotrauma, pulmonary: mechanical ventilation. CINAHL Nursing Guide. 2011. Glendale (CA): Cinahl Information Systems; 2011, Available at: http://search.ebscohost.com/login.aspx?direct=true&db=nrc&AN=5000003217&site=nrc-live.Accessed August 25, 2011.

41. Johnson MM, Ely EW, Chiles C, et al. Radiographic assessment of hyperinflation: correlation with objective chest radiographic measurements and mechanical ventilator parameters. Chest 1998;113:1698–704.

42. Lewis R. Cabrera G. Atelectasis: mechanical ventilation. CINAHL Nursing Guide. 2011. Glendale (CA): Cinahl Information Systems; 2011. Available at: http://search.ebscohost.com/login.aspx?direct=true&db=nrc&AN=5000003374&site=nrc-live. Accessed August 25, 2011.

43. Jauncey-Cooke JI, Bogossian F, East CE. Lung recruitment—a guide for clinicians. Aust Crit Care 2009;22:155–62.

44. Papadakos PJ, Lachmann B, Koch R. Lung recruitment: a role in mechanical ventilation. Canadian Journal of Respiratory Therapy 2010;46:33–7.

45. Curley GF, Kevin LG, Laffey JG. Mechanical ventilation: taking its toll on the lung. Anesthesiology 2009;111:701–3.

46. Hegeman MA, Hennus MP, Heijnen CJ, et al. Ventilator-induced endothelial activation and inflammation in the lung and distal organs. Crit Care 2009;13:R182. Available at: http://www.ncbi.nlm.nih.gov/pmc/articles/PMC2811914/. Accessed August 25, 2011.

47. LaFollette R, Hojnowski K, Norton J, et al. Using pressure-volume curves to set proper PEEP in acute lung injury. Nurs Crit Care 2007;12:231–41.

48. Kuebler WM. From a distance: ventilation-dependent extra-pulmonary injury. Transl Res 2010;155:217–9.

Electrolyte Disorders in the Cardiac Patient

Carol Hinkle, MSN, RN-BC

KEYWORDS

- Electrolytes • Electrocardiographic changes
- Electrolyte disorders • Hyperkalemia • Hypokalemia
- Hypomagnesemia

Electrolytes are important for many functions of the body.[1] Disorders of these electrolytes can cause multiple problems for cardiac patients. Many patients have comorbidities such as renal insufficiency that affect electrolyte balance as well. This article will discuss electrolyte function in the heart and electrolyte disorders that can cause problems for the heart. There will also be a brief discussion of patient problems that can alter electrolyte balance.

Electrolytes perform a variety of functions in the human body.[2,3] The body, primarily the kidney, maintains electrolytes within a narrow physiologic range.[4] Disorders may involve either too little (hypo-) or too much (hyper-) of specific electrolytes. The functioning heart is dependent on normal levels of calcium, magnesium, phosphorus, potassium, and sodium.[2,5] The electrical activity of the heart is controlled by calcium, potassium, and sodium, whereas contraction of the heart requires calcium, magnesium, and phosphorus.[2,5] Calcium is important in initiating the excitation-contraction coupling.[2,5,6] These electrolytes are all necessary for the electrical and mechanical operation of the heart.

ELECTROLYTE FUNCTIONS

Potassium is the electrolyte that most people associate with the heart. It is the major intracellular cation and functions to maintain osmolality and electroneutrality inside the cell.[7,8] Potassium can also exchange with hydrogen ions to assist in maintaining acid-base balance.[3,7] Potassium maintains the transmembrane action potential and is important in both impulse formation and conduction.[7,9] Interestingly, it seems that the atrial cell is more sensitive to changes in potassium than the ventricular cell.[10]

Calcium has many important functions in the heart. It helps to maintain cell wall integrity and cell permeability.[3,11] Ringer was the first to realize the importance of calcium on the contraction of the heart.[12] We now know that calcium assists in the actin-myosin

The author has nothing to disclose.

Education Consultant–Critical Care, Education Department, Brookwood Medical Center, 2010 Medical Center Drive, Birmingham, AL 35209, USA

E-mail address: Carol.Hinkle@tenethealth.com

Crit Care Nurs Clin N Am 23 (2011) 635–643

doi:10.1016/j.ccell.2011.08.008

cross bridge necessary for myocardial cell contraction.[6] According to Stark, major functions of calcium are "generation of cardiac action potential and pacemaker function."[8] Potter and Perry mention calcium's role in cardiac conduction.[1]

Phosphorus is another intracellular anion that is important for the heart. The term phosphorus is generally used interchangeably with phosphate.[1] It is mostly involved in intracellular energy production with its role in the formation of adenosine triphosphate (ATP).[11,13] Phosphorus is important in promoting the "release of oxygen within the cell."[13] Phosphates also assist in maintaining the integrity of the myocardial cell membrane.[3]

Magnesium, the second most abundant intracellular cation after potassium, has many varied functions in relation to the heart.[14] Magnesium is important in the cell's biochemical reactions. Some of magnesium's benefits to the heart may include enhanced coronary blood flow, conservation of potassium, improved myocardial cell function, and decreased arrhythmias.[8] Innerarity reports that "magnesium functions to produce peripheral vasodilation, which results in changes in blood pressure and cardiac output."[13] Potter and Perry state that magnesium is important for cardiac muscle excitability.[1]

Sodium is well known as the major extracellular cation that significantly affects fluid balance in patients. Sodium assists in the exchange of water between intracellular and extracellular spaces in the body and is a major component in the measurement of the body's serum osmolality.[1,11,15] Sodium is important for the depolarization and repolarization of cells because of its role in the action potential.[5,15]

CARDIAC EFFECTS DUE TO ELECTROLYTE DISORDERS

Electrolyte disorders can cause changes to the normal electrocardiogram (ECG) (**Table 1**). Many of these changes can also be caused by conditions other than abnormal electrolytes.[6] Therefore, the patient's ECG must always be viewed within the context of the overall picture including the results of serum electrolytes. Electrolyte disorders cause other changes to patients that can affect the heart. Many times, patients are experiencing more than one electrolyte disorder at the same time, which further complicates their care.[1]

Sodium, by itself, does not have direct effects on the heart or the cardiovascular system. However, because of the effects of sodium on the body's fluid balance, we see many effects. If the fluid balance is decreased, the patient may exhibit tachycardia, hypotension, and a decreased central venous pressure (CVP). Conversely, if the fluid balance is increased, the patient may have hypertension, elevated CVP, and jugular venous distention.[8] The patient with hypernatremia who also has weight gain may show signs of peripheral edema, or, even worse, pulmonary edema due to heart failure.[16] Atrial natriuretic peptide is released in the heart when the patient has volume overload and stretching of the atria.[2,6] This peptide causes the kidneys to increase excretion of sodium and this increases the excretion of water, which will decrease volume in the body.

Cardiac patients can have problems with fluid volume overload, especially after acute myocardial infarction (MI) with left ventricular dysfunction or patients who are admitted with congestive heart failure (CHF).[4,16] Additionally, many patients, particularly the elderly, may be dehydrated upon admission to a critical care unit. Fluid volume overload or dehydration may affect the patient's sodium levels.

There are many studies linking the increased dietary intake of sodium to an increase in blood pressure, which is a major preventable risk factor for both coronary artery disease and stroke. Many people with an increased intake of sodium also have a decreased intake of potassium and magnesium, which has been reported to have

Table 1
Effects of electrolyte disorders

Disorder	ECG Changes	Other Cardiac Effects
Hypokalemia $K^+ < 3.5$ mEq/L	Ventricular dysrhythmias Flat or inverted T wave Presence of U wave QT or QU prolongation ST segment depression Blending of T and U wave	Enhanced digitalis effect Bradycardia Premature atrial contractions AV blocks

Hyperkalemia
$K^+ > 5.5$ mEq/L
	Peaked, elevated T wave with
	  narrow base
	Prolongation of PR interval
	Flattened P wave that may
	  disappear
	Widened QRS complex
	Sine wave due to QRS and T
	  wave combining
		Bradycardia
		First degree AV block
		Hypotension
		Progresses to ventricular
		  fibrillation or ventricular
		  standstill

Hypocalcemia $Ca^{++} < 8.5$ mg/dl	Prolonged ST segment Prolonged QT interval Flattened or inverted T wave	Dysrhythmias Irregular pulse
Hypercalcemia $Ca^{++} > 10.5$ mg/dl	Shortened QT interval Shortened ST segments that may appear sagging Inverted T wave	Hypertension Ventricular dysrhythmias Enhanced digitalis effect
Hypomagnesemia $Mg^{++} < 1.5$ mEq/L	Flattened or inverted T wave Depression of ST segment Prolonged QT interval	Ventricular dysrhythmias Enhanced digitalis effect
Hypermagnesemia $Mg^{++} > 2.2$ mEq/L	Peaked T wave Prolonged PR interval	Bradycardia Hypotension

Abbreviation: ECG, Electrocardiogram.

a protective effect on the heart. Increasing dietary potassium has been shown to cause a fall in blood pressure in both hypertensive and normotensive people and is associated with a decreased incidence of stroke.[17]

Signs and symptoms of magnesium imbalance are frequently mistaken for calcium imbalance because they are similar.[13,16] Therefore, it is best to monitor the patient's electrolyte levels to determine which imbalances are present. Hypermagnesemia can lead to serious cardiac problems.[4,14] Because of its effect as a calcium channel blocker, hypermagnesemia causes peripheral vasodilation leading to hypotension.[13] It is important to monitor patients with hypermagnesemia for increased PR interval and the development of complete heart block.[4] Hypermagnesemia has a depressant effect on skeletal muscle and nerve function, which decreases acetylcholine levels and leads to decreased respiratory rate and depth, bradycardia, and eventually cardiac arrest.[1] The emergent treatment of hypermagnesemia uses calcium gluconate intravenously to decrease the depressant effects of magnesium.[4,16] Dextrose 50% and intravenous (IV) regular insulin may offer a temporary fix by forcing magnesium back into the cell.[13] If the hypermagnesemia is not too severe, fluids and diuretics can be used if the patient's renal function is not impaired; otherwise, dialysis may be required to remove the magnesium.[4]

Hypomagnesemia leads to increased cardiac excitability, although it is believed that the primary cause of premature ventricular contractions may be due to a failure to maintain intracellular potassium levels.[11,14] A decrease in the serum magnesium may enhance the effects of digitalis.[8] In addition to causing hypertension in some patients, hypomagnesemia can lead to coronary and cerebral artery spasms.[13,18] Hypomagnesemia can be treated with replacement therapy. However, if the patient has both low magnesium and low potassium levels, the magnesium level needs to be corrected first because of magnesium's role in the functioning of the cell's sodium-potassium pump.[16]

It has been reported that magnesium administration during an acute MI may decrease mortality by 24% and improve ventricular function by 25%.[8] In the early 1970s, Anderson and colleagues reported on the potential effects of decreased magnesium levels in water on the increased incidence of ischemic heart disease and sudden cardiac death in populations, stating that "relatively high death rates in some soft-water areas may be due to a suboptimal intake of magnesium, and . . . water-borne magnesium exerts a protective effect on the residents of hard-water areas."[19]

In the 1990s, there were conflicting research reports about IV magnesium decreasing the incidence of ventricular arrhythmias. Currently, the American College of Cardiology/American Heart Association guidelines recommend correcting documented magnesium deficiencies, especially in patients receiving diuretics before onset of ST elevation MI (class IIa).[6] They also recommend that episodes of torsades de pointes–type ventricular tachycardia associated with a prolonged QT interval should be treated with IV magnesium (class IIa).[6]

The range of serum potassium (3.5–5.5 mEq/L) is very small; therefore, the tolerance of the body for changes is also small.[1,7] The most common causes of hyperkalemia include: renal failure or insufficiency, certain medications, cardiac failure, insulin deficiency and metabolic acidosis, and the use of a salt substitute.[8,16] If the patient develops a sudden hyperkalemia, the nurse should consider the possibility of specimen hemolysis.[7,13] The blood specimen needs to be re-collected if this is a possibility. Common causes of hypokalemia include: thiazide and loop diuretics, gastrointestinal (GI) losses (nasogastric suction, vomiting, or diarrhea), kidneys unable to concentrate urine, increased aldosterone levels causing sodium to be reabsorbed and potassium excreted, and osmotic diuresis in diabetic ketoacidosis (DKA).[8,13,16]

Many patients with cardiac problems may also have renal problems. This generally leads to hyperkalemia either due to the presence of chronic or acute renal failure. Patients with heart failure typically have decreased renal perfusion that can lead to increased potassium levels. These patients may also have increased levels of atrial natriuretic peptide, which causes the patient to lose sodium through the kidneys and retain potassium.[6] A large number of cardiac patients also have diabetes. If they have uncontrolled diabetes and develop DKA, the resultant metabolic acidosis initiates the exchange of potassium ions out of the cell and hydrogen ions into the cell, causing hyperkalemia.[13,16] Patients receiving diuretics for hypertension may develop hyperkalemia if they are administered potassium-sparing diuretics.[8]

The emergent treatment for severe hyperkalemia (K^+ >6.5 mEq/L) may include the administration of IV insulin and dextrose with a beta agonist (ie, inhaled albuterol) or IV sodium bicarbonate.[4,8] This treatment temporarily drives potassium into the cell until definitive treatment is started. The definitive treatment may include the administration of kayexalate or a dialysis treatment.[4] If the hyperkalemia is causing serious cardiac arrhythmias such as bradycardia progressing to asystole, administering IV calcium gluconate or calcium chloride will help to stabilize the cell membrane.[8]

Some commonly used medications can lead to hypokalemia. These include loop and thiazide diuretics, gentamycin, dopamine, epinephrine, and norepinephrine.[8,13] Also, because severe stress increases the levels of epinephrine and norepinephrine in the body, this can also lead to decreased potassium levels.[8] Any patient with a high urine output or increased GI losses should be suspected of losing potassium as well.[16] Potassium levels can fluctuate in patients who are receiving insulin. The higher the dose of insulin, the lower the potassium level may be.[7,13] Also, although DKA initially causes an elevated potassium level, hypokalemia soon develops because of the osmotic diuresis.[4,13] Therefore, the nurse should always keep a close check on the patient's most recent laboratory values, particularly their potassium.

Patients with hypokalemia are at increased risk for developing ventricular dysrhythmias.[4,16] It is believed that a low potassium level alters the cell's resting membrane potential, leading to increased excitability of the cell. It is a well-known fact that hypokalemia enhances the effects of digitalis, even leading to toxicity.[8] Therefore, it is recommended that cardiac monitoring be initiated for those patients who are suspected of having a potassium imbalance.[16] Hypokalemia is easily corrected with an IV infusion of potassium.[4]

Calcium and phosphorus are generally in an inverse proportion.[11,13] That is, if the calcium is low, the phosphorus is high and vice versa. The most common cause of calcium or phosphorus imbalances is renal failure, either acute or chronic.[8,16] In renal failure, phosphorus is not excreted and this leads to a decrease in calcium. Also, the active form of vitamin D is unavailable, which means that dietary sources of calcium are not absorbed, leading to hypocalcemia during renal failure.[13] The administration of corticosteroids can decrease the GI absorption of calcium.[8] Also, the nurse should check the patient's albumin levels because 50% of calcium can be bound to albumin. If the patient is diuresing after an episode of acute renal failure or receiving diuretics, phosphorus, potassium, and magnesium are lost.[13]

In addition to ECG changes related to imbalances of calcium, the nurse should be observant for arrhythmias. It is possible to see ventricular tachycardia with hypocalcemia.[16] Because of the role of calcium in the clotting cascade, hypocalcemia may lead to increased clotting times and potentially bleeding.[11,13] Hypercalcemia can lead to the development of atrioventricular block progressing to cardiac arrest but may also cause tachycardia or paroxysmal atrial tachycardia.[11,13] Hypercalcemia can lead to an enhanced digitalis effect if the patient is receiving this medication.[16] The nurse may find hypertension in about 33% of patients with hypercalcemia.[8] Hypophosphatemia can cause arrhythmias and lead to a cardiomyopathy due to a decrease in stroke volume.[16] Hyperphosphatemia does not cause specific cardiac problems.

The treatment of hypocalcemia or hypophosphatemia usually involves replacement therapy either orally or intravenously depending on the severity of the imbalance.[4] Dietary counseling is important as part of the patient's discharge planning. Hypercalcemia may be treated with diuretics and fluids if renal status is normal. This may involve 4 to 6 L of normal saline solution over a 12-hour period.[16] Or, if the patient is able, he or she may ingest 3 to 4 L of fluids per day. Hyperphosphatemia is usually treated with phosphate binders. In the emergency situation, dialysis may be required.

ELECTROLYTE DISORDERS IN THE CARDIAC SURGICAL PATIENT

It is well known that patients who undergo cardiac surgery with extracorporeal circulation are at high risk for electrolyte depletion.[18] In practice, most post-surgical protocols check potassium levels more frequently than other electrolytes. Polderman and Girbes recommend that "magnesium, potassium, phosphate and calcium be frequently measured during and after cardiac surgery."[18]

Some of the specific problems seen in patients who are post bypass include: cardiac arrhythmias with hypokalemia; increased mortality, cardiac arrhythmias, hypertension and vasoconstriction (including the coronary arteries) with hypomagnesemia; arrhythmias with shortening of the QT interval, cardiovascular depression and CHF with hypocalcemia; low levels of ATP leading to muscle weakness, respiratory failure, decrease in cardiac output, and ventricular tachycardia with hypophosphatemia.[18,20–22] The mechanism for the lowering of electrolyte levels during cardiopulmonary bypass appears to be hypothermia-induced diuresis and intracellular shifts. This occurs despite using cardioplegia solutions containing both potassium and magnesium.[18] Therefore, more frequent monitoring of electrolytes in cardiac surgery patients should be considered.

CONDITIONS CAUSING ELECTROLYTE DISTURBANCES IN CARDIAC PATIENTS

It has already been stated that electrolyte disorders rarely occur either singly or in isolation. This means that it is common to see several disorders at the same time, and that many patients with an admitting diagnosis for something other than electrolyte disorder will exhibit this problem also. In fact, there are several diagnoses when the nurse should suspect an electrolyte problem. These include dehydration or volume overload, acidosis of various etiologies, nutrition issues, renal or liver disease, heart failure, and pancreatitis. Also, there are certain classes of medications that frequently lead to electrolyte disorders. These can include diuretics (the major culprit), angiotensin-converting enzyme inhibitors, angiotensin II antagonists, beta blockers, calcium channel blockers, some antibiotics, nonsteroidal antiinflammatory drugs, vasoactive medications such as dopamine, epinephrine, or norepinephrine, and heparin. Other issues such as prolonged bed rest or severe stress can also lead to electrolyte disorders. Cardiac monitoring is indicated for patients with electrolyte disorders.[23]

Cardiovascular risk and renal risk occur together in many of our patients. McCullough states that "the heart and kidney are. . .linked in terms of hemodynamic and regulatory functions."[24] According to the US Renal Data System, cardiovascular disease is the number one cause of death in patients with end-stage renal disease undergoing dialysis.[25] Castellanos and colleagues state that "chronic renal insufficiency has been independently associated with. . .cardiovascular events."[6] Many cardiovascular risk factors or symptoms are also associated with renal problems. These include hypertension, diabetes, obesity, and volume overload.

Any patient with an admitting diagnosis of chronic renal failure or chronic renal insufficiency or who develops a new acute renal failure is certainly going to have electrolyte disorders.[26] Because the kidney is the major regulator of electrolyte levels in the body, any disruption in kidney function alters electrolytes.[4] Most of the electrolyte levels will be elevated if the kidney is unable to clear them from the body; however, the nurse should expect calcium levels to be decreased. On the other hand, if the patient is experiencing an increase in urine output or is taking diuretics, many electrolytes will be lost with the urine including calcium. Also, many of the electrolyte levels will appear low during fluid volume overload because of a dilutional effect.[16] This is particularly true of a dilutional hyponatremia.

Patients admitted with CHF have many problems with electrolyte disorders. Most of these patients have problems with volume overload and are taking diuretics that can alter electrolyte levels as discussed previously. Many patients with CHF can have a decreased cardiac output that affects renal perfusion and can cause electrolyte levels to fluctuate. We are also learning about the role of natriuretic peptides in patients with CHF.[6,15,16] This peptide is released in response to atrial distention (as in volume overload due to heart failure) and has 2 effects. It promotes vasodilation and natriuresis, which increases sodium excretion through the kidneys.[6] Therefore, electrolyte levels may be abnormal.

Acidosis can be caused by many different patient problems. During an acidosis, electrolytes can move out of the cell (called a transmembrane shift) to exchange with the high levels of hydrogen ions in the body.[7,13,16] This can cause the serum concentrations of these electrolytes to appear falsely elevated. This shift appears in patients with diabetic ketoacidosis or lactic acidosis. Also, acute renal failure frequently causes a metabolic acidosis because of the kidney's inability to get rid of excess hydrogen ions.[4] Any time that the patient's pH is less than 7.30, it is a good idea to check electrolyte levels.

Many GI problems can also affect the body's electrolyte balance. Electrolytes can be lost during nasogastric suction, vomiting, or diarrhea.[12] Malnutrition can certainly contribute to electrolyte disorders because these substances are ingested as part of a normal diet.[7] Pancreatitis is another illness that is frequently associated with disorders of the patient's electrolytes. Hypocalcemia and hypomagnesemia are frequently seen during acute pancreatitis.[4]

SUMMARY

In conclusion, electrolyte disorders are common in cardiovascular patients and complicate the care of these patients. The vigilant nurse expects electrolyte abnormalities in their patients and assesses for signs and symptoms related to them. The symptomatology of electrolyte disorders can be vague or the patient's symptoms may have multiple causes. Therefore, the nurse should always assess for the most recent laboratory work available for patients and be alert for changes in electrolyte values. Cardiac monitoring is indicated for these patients because many electrolyte disorders can contribute to cardiac arrhythmias or may cause electrocardiographic changes.

ACKNOWLEDGMENTS

I would like to thank Charlene Roberson for drawings and Shawn Cosper for assistance.

REFERENCES

1. Potter P, Perry A, editors. Fluid, electrolyte, and acid-bace balances in fundamentals of nursing. 6th edition. St. Louis: Elsevier Mosby; 2005. p. 1135–97.
2. Berl T, Schrier RW. Disorders of water homeostasis. In: Schrier RW, editor. Renal and electrolyte disorders. 7th edition. Philadelphia: Wolters Kluwer; 2010. p. 1–44.
3. Innerarity SA. Fluids and electrolytes. Philadelphia: Lippincott Williams Wilkins; 1997.
4. Hinkle C. Renal system. In: Chulay M, Burns SM, editors. AACN Essentials of Critical Care Nursing. 2nd edition. New York: McGraw Hill, 2010. p. 357–71.
5. Fisch C. Electrolytes and the heart. In: Hurst JW, Logue RB, Rackley CE, et al, editors. The heart. 5th edition. New York: McGraw Hill; 1982. p. 1599–611.
6. Castellanos A, Interian A, Myerburg RJ. The resting electrocardiogram. In: Fuster V, Alexander RW, O'Rourke RA, et al, editors. Hurst's the heart. 11th edition. New York: McGraw-Hill Book Co; 2004. p. 295–324.
7. Palmer BF, Dubose TD. Disorders of potassium metabolism In: Schrier RW, editor. Renal and electrolyte disorders. 7th edition. Philadelphia: Wolters Kluwer; 2010. p. 137–65.
8. Stark JL. The renal system. In: Alspach JG, editor. Core curriculum for critical care nursing. 6th edition. Philadelphia: Elsevier Saunders, 2006. p. 525–602.
9. Fisch C. Relation of electrolyte disturbances to cardiac arrhythmias. Circulation 1973;47:408–19.
10. Hoffman BF, Cranefield PF. Electrophysiology of the heart. New York: McGraw-Hill Book Co, 1960.
11. Popovtzer MM. Disorders of calcium, phosphorus, vitamin D, and parathyroid hormone activity. In: Schrier RW, editors. Renal and electrolyte disorders. 7th edition. Philadelphia: Wolters Kluwer; 2010. p. 166–228.
12. Ringer S. A further contribution regarding the influence of the different constituents of blood on the contraction of the heart. J Physiol 1183;4:29.
13. Innerarity SA. Electrolyte emergencies in the critically ill renal patient. Crit Care Nurs Clin North Am 1990;2:89–99.
14. Spiegel DM. Normal and abnormal magnesium metabolism. In: Schrier RW, editor. Renal and electrolyte disorders. 7th edition. Philadelphia: Wolters Kluwer; 2010. p. 229–50.
15. Schrier RW. Renal sodium excretion, edematous disorders, and diuretic use. Renal and electrolyte disorders. 7th edition. Philadelphia: Wolters Kluwer; 2010. p. 45–85.
16. Horne MM, Bond EF. Fluid, electrolyte, and acid-base imbalances. In: Medical-Surgical Nursing: Assessment and Management of Clinical Problems. 5th edition. St. Louis: Mosby; 2000. p. 323–50.
17. National Heart Foundation of Australia. The relationships between dietary electrolytes and cardiovascular disease, 2006. Available at: http://www.heartfoundation.com.au. Accessed September 5, 2011.
18. Polderman KH, Girbes AR. Severe electrolyte disorders following cardiac surgery: a prospective controlled observational study. Crit Care 2004;8:R459–66.
19. Anderson TW, Neri LC, Schreiber GB, et al. Ischemic heart disease, water hardness and myocardial magnesium. Can Med Assoc J 1975;113:199–203.
20. Stelfox HT, Ahmed SB, Zygun D, et al. Characterization of intensive care unit acquired hyponatremia and hypernatremia following cardiac surgery. Can J Anesth 2010;57: 650–8.
21. Pasternak K, Dabrowski W, Dobija J, et al. The effect of preoperative magnesium supplementation on blood catecholamine concentrations in patients undergoing CABG. Magnes Res 2006;19:113–22.

22. Baker WL, Whit CM. Post-cardiothoracic surgery atrial fibrillation: review of preventative strategies. Ann Pharmacother 2007;41;587–98.

23. Chen EH, Hollander JE. When do patients need admission to a telemetry bed? J Emerg Med 2007;33:53–60.

24. McCullough P. Interface Between Renal Disease and Cardiovascular Illness. In: Zipes DP, Libby P, Bonow RP, et al, editors. Braunwald's heart disease: a textbook of cardiovascular medicine. 7th edition. Philadelphia: Elsevier Saunders, 2005. p. 2161–72.

25. US Renal Data System, USRDS 2010 Annual Data Report: Atlas of chronic kidney disease and end-stage renal disease in the United States. Bethesda (MD): National Institutes of Health, National Institute of Diabetes and Digestive and Kidney Diseases; 2010.

26. Schrier RW, Edelstein CL. Acute kidney injury: pathogenesis, diagnosis, and management. In: Schrier RW.Renal and electrolyte disorders.7th edition. Philadelphia: Wolters Kluwer; 2010. p. 325–88.

Pulmonary Arterial Hypertension

Mae M. Centeno, DNP, RN, CCRN, CCNS, ACNS-BC

KEYWORDS

- Pulmonary hypertension • Pulmonary arterial hypertension
- Classification • Medical Treatment
- Pharmacologic Intervention

Pulmonary arterial hypertension (PAH) is a rare disease, with an estimated prevalence of 30 to 50 cases per million.[1] The prevalence of PAH varies and may even be higher in certain at-risk groups. Data collected by the National Institute of Health Registry from 1981 to 1985 reported a median survival of 2.8 years with survival rates 68%, 48%, and 34% after 1, 3, and 5 years, respectively.[2] PAH is a diagnosis of exclusion. Patients usually present in the advance stage of the disease, suggesting the true prevalence may be higher than what is in the literature.[1] This article provides an insightful and helpful review of the classification of pulmonary hypertension, assessment, and treatment options.

DEFINITION

Pulmonary hypertension (PH) is a complex, chronic disorder causing an elevation in pulmonary artery pressures. The suspicion and detection of PH requires a comprehensive diagnostic workup to determine hemodynamic profile and possible causes.[3] PAH is a category of PH (Dana Point Group 1) (**Table 1**).[4] Pulmonary hypertension and PAH are 2, nonsynonymous terms.[5] PAH refers to the presence of a mean pulmonary artery pressure exceeding 25 mm Hg, a normal pulmonary capillary wedge pressure of 15 mm Hg or less, and a pulmonary vascular resistance of greater than 3 wood units.[3] The determination of hemodynamics is through an invasive evaluation by right heart catheterization.

CLASSIFICATION OF PULMONARY HYPERTENSION

The classification of PH has undergone various revisions since the first classification was proposed in 1973.[4] The initial classification had 2 categories, primary PH or secondary PH based on the presence of risk factors or identifiable causes. Subsequent changes were made to the classification in an attempt to categorize

Speaker for Actelion, Gilead and United Therapeutics.
Heart Failure Program and Advanced Lung Disease Center, Baylor University Medical Center, 3500 Gaston Avenue, Dallas, TX 75246, USA
E-mail address: Mae.Centeno@Baylorhealth.edu

Crit Care Nurs Clin N Am 23 (2011) 645–659
doi:10.1016/j.ccell.2011.08.010
0899-5885/11/$ – see front matter © 2011 Elsevier Inc. All rights reserved.

Table 1
Updated clinical classification of pulmonary hypertension (Dana Point, 2008)

1. Pulmonary arterial hypertension (PAH)
    1.1. Idiopathic PAH
    1.2. Heritable
        1.2.1. BMPR2
        1.2.2. ALK$_1$ endoglin (with or without hereditary hemorrhagic telangectasia)
        1.2.3. Unknown
    1.3. Drug-and-toxin-induced
    1.4. Associated with
        1.4.1. Connective tissue disease
        1.4.2. HIV infection
        1.4.3. Portal hypertension
        1.4.4. Congenital heart disease
        1.4.5. Schistosomiasis
        1.4.6. Chronic hemolytic anemia
    1.5. Persistent pulmonary hypertension of the newborn
    1'. Pulmonary veno-occlusive disease (PVOD) and/or pulmonary capillary hemangiomatosis (PCH)

2. Pulmonary hypertension owing to left to left heart disease
    2.1. Systolic dysfunction
    2.2. Diastolic dysfunction
    2.3. Valvular disease

3. Pulmonary hypertension owing to lung disease and/or hypoxia
    3.1. Chronic obstructive pulmonary disease
    3.2. Interstitial lung disease
    3.3. Other pulmonary diseases with mixed restrictive and obstructive pattern
    3.4. Sleep-disordered breathing
    3.5. Alveolar hypoventilation orders
    3.6. Chronic exposure to high altitude
    3.7. Developmental abnormalities

4. Chronic thromboembolic pulmonary hypertension (CTEPH)

5. Pulmonary hypertension with unclear multifactorial mechanisms
    5.1. Hematologic disorders: myeloproliferative disorders, splenectomy
    5.2. Systemic disorders: Sarcoidosis, pulmonary Langerhans cell histiocytosis, lymphangiolelomyomatosis, neurofibromatosis, vasculitis
    5.3. Metabolic disorders: glycogen storage disease, Gaucher disease, thyroid disorders
    5.4. Others: tumoral obstruction, fibrosing mediastinitis, chronic renal failure on dialysis

Reprinted Simonneau G, Robbins IM, Beghetti M, et al. Updated clinical classification of pulmonary hypertension. J Am Coll Card 2009;54:S43–54; with permission.

PH based on pathologic and clinical features as well as treatment options.[6] In 2008, during the 4th World Symposium on PH in Dana Point, California, the classification of PH (see **Table 1**) was updated to reflect research published in the last 5 years.[4]

Table 2	
Updated risk factors for and associated conditions of PAH	
Definite	**Possible**
Aminorex	Cocaine
Fenfluramine	Phenylpropanolamine
Dexfenfluramine	St. John's Wort
Toxic rapeseed oil	Chemotherapeutic agents
	Selective serotonin reuptake inhibitor
Likely	**Unlikely**
Amphetamines	Oral contraceptives
L-tryptophan	Estrogen
Methamphetamines	Cigarette smoking

From Simonneau G, Robbins IM, Beghetti M, et al. Updated clinical classification of pulmonary hypertension. J Am Coll Card 2009;54:S43–54; with permission.

Group 1

PAH is the group that has been the focus since 1973.[4] Greater understanding of the characteristics of the diseases under this group influenced the development of currently available treatment options.

Idiopathic PAH is a rare disease without any identifiable risk factors, occurring in 1 per million.[7] It affects more women than men at the ratio of 1.7 to 1 with a mean age of 37 at the time of diagnosis.[8] Recent reports suggest that idiopathic pulmonary arterial hypertension (IPAH) occurs in patients older than 70 years.[9]

Heritable PAH, formerly familial PAH, occurs in approximately 6% to 10% of PAH cases.[5] It includes patients with germline mutations of bone morphogenic protein receptor type 2 (BMPR2) gene in approximately 70% of cases[10,11] and, rarely, activin receptor–like kinase 1 or endoglin.[4] Genetic testing is not mandated; however, when performed, it should include genetic counseling.[4]

Drug- and toxin-induced PAH was observed initially in the 1960s, after the introduction of aminorex fumarate, an appetite suppressant.[5,12] Use of drugs of similar structure, such as fenfluramine and dexfenfluramine, has been associated with increase risks of PAH.[5,13] Other drugs, such as rapeseed oil,[4,14] L-typtophan,[4,15] methamphetamine, and cocaine[4,16] have also been linked to the development of PAH. **Table 2** lists drugs with definite, possible, likely, and unlikely risk associated to development of PAH.[4]

PAH associated with connective tissue disease develops in approximately 10% of patients with systemic sclerosis.[4,17] PAH has been observed in systemic lupus erythematosus, rheumatoid arthritis, and mixed connective disease; however, the prevalence remains unknown. The echocardiogram is used as a screening tool for the development of PAH in these patients.[4,5]

PAH in patients with HIV has a prevalence of 0.5%, independent of CD4 count or prior opportunistic infections.[18] The mechanism for the development of PAH in human immunodeficiency virus (HIV) is not well understood, yet it remains a known complication.[4]

PAH associated with portal hypertension, known as *portopulmonary hypertension* (POPH), occurs in patients with cirrhosis at a rate of 2% to 6% and maybe higher in patients undergoing evaluation for liver transplant.[4,19] High flow states and left ventricular diastolic dysfunction in advanced liver disease may influence elevation of pulmonary artery pressures.[4] Right heart catheterization is required for a definitive diagnosis of POPH.[4]

PAH associated with congenital heart disease (CHD) is known as *Eisenmenger syndrome*. It occurs in approximately 25% to 50% of patients with untreated left-to-right shunt, such as ventricular septal defect, patent ductus arteriosus, or truncus arteriosus. The persistent exposure of the pulmonary vasculature to increased blood flow and pressure increases pulmonary vascular resistance leading to pulmonary hypertension, a right- to- left shunt and central cyanosis.[20]

PAH associated with schistosomiasis occurs in countries in which the infection is endemic.[4,21] The patients with schistosomiasis have similar clinical presentation to IPAH, reinforcing the need for proper diagnosis through heart catheterization.[4,21] Patients in whom hepatosplenic disease develops from schistosomiasis have a 4.6% incidence of PAH.[21]

PAH associated with hemolytic anemia is increasingly recognized in sickle cell disease, with a prevalence of 10% to 30% and a 2-year mortality rate of 50%.[22,23] Thromboembolic disease, restrictive lung disease, and left heart disease maybe contributing factors to PH in sickle disease.[23]

Persistent pulmonary hypertension of the newborn is characterized by severe hypoxemia, right-to-left shunt, and increased pulmonary vascular resistance.[4] Lack of endogenous nitric oxide and elevated endothelin levels have been documented in this population, with a mortality rate of 20%.[4]

Pulmonary veno-occlusive disease (PVOD) and pulmonary capillary hemangiomatosis (PCH) are difficult to categorize, as both present like IPAH.[24] The use of vasodilators, such as epoprostenol in PVOD or PCH, is associated with rapid development of pulmonary edema.[24]

Group 2

PH due to left heart disease (see **Table 1**) is caused by systolic dysfunction, diastolic dysfunction, or valvular heart disease.[4] The increase in left atrial pressure is reflected backward to the pulmonary veins, and backward pressure increases pulmonary artery pressures leading to pulmonary hypertension. The pulmonary vascular resistance remains less than 3 wood units and a transpulmonary gradient of less than 12 mm Hg. Pulmonary vascular resistance measures the resistance in the pulmonary vascular bed against which the right ventricle must eject blood. The transpulmonary gradient is the difference between the mean pulmonary artery pressure and the pulmonary capillary wedge pressure. Some patients have severe PH out of proportion to left heart disease. There are no data to suggest that approved medications for PAH are safe and efficacious in this population.[4]

Group 3

PH caused by lung disease or hypoxia is associated with various diseases (see **Table 1**) leading to inflammatory, fibrotic, and destruction of the lung parenchyma. The resulting alveolar hypoxia from lung disease is the predominant cause of PH. The prevalence of PH in these conditions remains unknown. In combined pulmonary fibrosis and emphysema, the prevalence is almost 50%.[25] As with PH out of proportion to left heart disease, medications approved for PAH are not available for PH out of proportion for lung disease.[4]

Group 4

Chronic thromboembolic pulmonary hypertension (CTEPH) affects 4% of patients after an acute pulmonary embolism.[26] Expert evaluation of patients with suspected or confirmed cases of CTEPH to assess the feasibility of undergoing pulmonary thromboendarterectomy, the only curative treatment, is highly recommended.[27] PAH-approved medical therapy may benefit patients who are not surgical candidates; however, use of these medications in CTEPH requires further evaluation.[28]

Group 5

PH with unclear or multifactorial etiologies (see **Table 1**) includes hematologic, systemic, and metabolic disorders and miscellaneous conditions.[4] The prevalence of PH is variable. A high degree of suspicion for PH is imperative to appropriately treat or refer these patients.[4]

PATHOLOGY

The pulmonary circulation is normally characterized by low pressure and low vascular resistance. The pulmonary arteries dilate and constrict to control pulmonary vascular resistance. In PAH, there is persistent elevation of pulmonary pressure leading to pulmonary artery vascular changes, such as chronic vasoconstriction, smooth muscle hypertrophy, and proliferation.[29] In addition, thrombosis secondary to endothelial dysfunction is observed. The presence of plexiform lesions, a result of intimal and adventitial proliferation, is present in advanced stages of PAH.[29] The altered pulmonary vascular endothelium causes an imbalance in prostacyclin, which causes vasodilation, and thromboxane, which causes vasoconstriction.[29] Furthermore, there is an overexpression of endothelin, a potent vasoconstrictor, and an impaired synthesis of the endothelium-derived nitric oxide, which causes vasodilation.[29] These vascular changes lead to a continuous increase in pulmonary artery pressures, impairing the right ventricular emptying, decreasing cardiac output, and eventually developing into right-sided heart failure.

EVALUATION PROCESS

The evaluation and management of patients with PH include suspicion in at-risk and symptomatic patients; screening; detecting and confirming the presence of PH; defining the hemodynamic state; identifying underlying cause or associated conditions; and determining prognosis, disease severity, and appropriate treatment.[30] Initial signs and symptoms are nonspecific, particularly in the early stages of the disease, resulting in delay in diagnosis of more than 2 years.[29]

The initial signs and symptoms of PAH reflect decreased oxygen availability and eventually reduce cardiac output, which includes shortness of breath, dyspnea on exertion, syncope, and chest pain related to right ventricular ischemia.[3] Physical findings depend on how advanced the disease is and may include accentuated pulmonary component of S_2, pulmonary outflow murmur, and a right ventricular heave. Advanced disease with right-sided heart failure signs includes jugular venous distention, peripheral edema, ascites, and right ventricular S_3.[5] The features of physical examination pertinent to the evaluation of PH are presented in **Table 3**. There are no signs and symptoms specific to PAH. Additional tests are required to confirm the diagnosis.

Multiple diagnostic tests are needed to appropriately evaluate a patient with PAH. Chest x-ray may show enlarged main pulmonary artery and right ventricular enlargement.[3] Electrocardiogram findings suggestive of PAH include right axis deviation, right ventricular strain, and right ventricular hypertrophy.[3] An echocardiogram raises the suspicion of PH and permits insight into the presence or absence of left ventricular dysfunction and valvular heart disease. Congenital heart disease and presence or

Table 3
Features of the physical examination pertinent to the evaluation of PH

Sign	Implication
Physical Signs that Reflect Severity of PH	
Accentuated pulmonary component	High pulmonary pressure increase force of pulmonic of S_2 (Audible at apex in over 90%) valve closure
Early systolic click	Sudden interruption of opening of pulmonary valve into high-pressure artery
Mid-systolic ejection murmur	Turbulent transvalvular pulmonary outflow
Left parasternal lift	High right ventricular pressure and hypertrophy present
Right ventricular S_4 (in 38%)	High right ventricular pressure and hypertrophy present
Increase jugular "a" wave	Poor right ventricular compliance
Physical Signs that Suggest Moderate to Severe PH	
Moderate to severe PH	
Holosystolic murmur that increases with inspiration	Tricuspid regurgitation
Increased jugular v waves	
Pulsatile liver	
Diastolic murmur	Pulmonary regurgitation
Hepatojugular reflux	High central venous pressure
Advanced PH with right ventricular failure	
Right ventricular S_3 (in 23%)	Right ventricular dysfunction
Distention of jugular veins	Right ventricular dysfunction or tricuspid regurgitation or both
Hepatomegaly	Right ventricular dysfunction or tricuspid regurgitation or both
Peripheral edema (in 32%)	
Ascites	
Low blood pressure, diminishedpulse pressure, cool extremities	Reduced cardiac output, peripheral vasoconstriction

Physical Sings that Suggest Possible Underlying Cause or Association of PH

Central cyanosis	Abnormal V/Q, intrapulmonary shunt, hypoxemia, Pulmonary-to-systemic shunt
Clubbing	Congenital heart disease, pulmonary venopathy
Cardiac auscultatory findings, including systolic murmurs, diastolicmurmurs, opening snap, and gallop	Congenital or acquired heart or valvular disease
Rales, dullness, or decreased breath sounds	Pulmonary congestion or effusion or both
Fine rales, accessory muscle use, wheezing, protracted expiration, productive cough	Pulmonary parenchymal disease
Obesity, kyphoscoliosis, enlarged tonsils	Possible substrate for disordered ventilation
Sclerodactyly, arthritis, telangiectasia, Raynaud phenomenon, rash	Connective tissue disorder
Peripheral venous insufficiency or obstruction	Possible venous thrombosis
Venous stasis ulcers	Possible sickle cell disease
Pulmonary vascular bruits	Chronic thromboembolic PH
Splenomegaly, spider angiomata, Palmary erythema, icterus, caput medusa, ascites	Portal hypertension

From McLaughlin VV, Archer SL, Badesch DB, et al. ACCF/AHA 2009 Expert consensus document on pulmonary hypertension: a report of the American College of Cardiology Foundation Task Force on Expert Consensus Documents and the American Heart Association developed in collaboration with the American College of Chest Physicians; American Thoracic Society, Inc.; and the Pulmonary Hypertension Association. J Am Coll Cardiol 2009; 53;1573–619; with permission.

absence of shunts can also be detected.[3] In addition, the echocardiogram provides estimated right ventricular systolic pressures suggestive of right atrial or right ventricular enlargement that are useful in predicting the severity of the disease.[3] Serial echocardiograms are beneficial in long-term follow-up to monitor response to treatment as well as disease progression. Echocardiograms do not confirm the diagnosis of PAH.[3]

Ventilation-perfusion scintigraphy is a highly sensitive test used to screen for chronic thromboembolic disease.[31] Pulmonary angiography is indicated if the ventilation-perfusion scintigraphy shows segmental or large perfusion defects.[3] High resolution computed tomography maybe used in place of ventilation perfusion studies. It is useful in patients with interstitial lung disease or pulmonary hypertension associated with connective tissue disease.[3] Pulmonary function tests are useful in detecting disorders such as restrictive or obstructive lung disease that maybe causing unexplained shortness of breath.[3] Overnight oximetry or sleep study should be done to detect the presence of sleep apnea and nocturnal hypoxemia, which may contribute to or exacerbate PH.[3] The 6-minute walk (6MW) is a simple, standardized exercise test to measure functional capacity, used to assess patients' responses to therapy and or disease progression.[3] In addition, the patients' functional abilities are graded using the World Health Organization functional classification.[32] It links symptoms with activity limitations and allows clinicians to quickly and accurately predict disease prognosis and assess disease progression during follow-up. Additional serologic tests to detect human immunodeficiency virus, hepatitis, and collagen vascular disease must be performed.[29]

Right heart catheterization measures pulmonary artery pressure, cardiac output, and pulmonary vascular resistance, which are necessary to confirm PAH diagnosis and exclude other secondary etiologies.[3] During catheterization, acute vasodilator testing is performed to assess the patient's response to short-acting vasodilators, such as inhaled nitric oxide, intravenous adenosine, and intravenous epoprostenol (**Table 4**).[5] Vasodilator testing must be performed in all patients with IPAH who may be considered potential candidates for calcium channel blockers. Vasodilator testing may be harmful and is not recommended in patients with significantly elevated filling pressures.[5] A positive response to vasodilator test occurs in 12.6% of patients[32] and

Table 4			
Agents for acute vasodilator testing			
	Epoprostenol	**Adenosine**	**Nitric Oxide**
Route of administration	Intravenous infusion	Intravenous infusion	Inhaled
Dose titration	2 ng/kg/min every 10–15 min	50 μg/kg/min every 2 min	None
Dose range	2–10 ng/kg/min	50–250 μg/kg/min	10 to 80 ppm
Side effects	Headache, nausea, lightheadedness	Dyspnea, chest pain, atrioventricular block	Increased left heart filling pressure in susceptible patients

From McLaughlin VV, Archer SL, Badesch DB, et al. ACCF/AHA 2009 Expert consensus document on pulmonary hypertension: A report of the American College of Cardiology Foundation Task Force on Expert Consensus Documents and the American Heart Association developed in collaboration with the American College of Chest Physicians; American Thoracic Society, Inc.; and the Pulmonary Hypertension Association. J Am Coll Cardiol 2009;53;1573–619; with permission.

is defined as a decrease in mean pulmonary arterial pressure of at least 10 mm Hg to an absolute mean pulmonary arterial pressure of less than 40 mm Hg without a decrease in cardiac output.[5] Positive responders are treated with calcium blockers with regular follow-up to reassess efficacy of therapy.[32]

MEDICAL TREATMENT

Treatment for PAH has evolved in the last decade because of a greater understanding of disease pathology as well as increased availability of medications targeting known deranged pathways. Treatment goals in PAH include improvement in symptoms, enhancing ability to perform daily activities, lowering pulmonary artery pressures, and normalizing cardiac output.[5] Another important goal is to prevent disease progression and prevent the need for more therapies, hospitalization, and lung transplantation.[5]

Low-impact exercise, such as walking, must be encouraged. It can improve 6MW, functional class, and quality of life. Heavy activities must be avoided because of the risk of exertional syncope.[33] The need for oxygen must be assessed because hypoxemia is a potent vasoconstrictor.[34] Oxygen supplementation to maintain oxygen saturation greater than 90% is recommended.[5] Patients with a preflight oxygen saturation of less than 92% should receive oxygen during their flight.[35] Patients may need resources on how to find out airline's policy on oxygen in flight. A sodium-restricted diet is important to manage fluid status in patients with right ventricular failure. Education on how to read food labels as well as how to make better food choices must be provided to patients and families. General measures to promote wellness such as hand washing and immunizations are encouraged.[5]

Pregnancy in patients with PAH carries a maternal mortality rate of 30% to 50%.[36] Patients must be counseled on the need for 2 forms of contraceptives and monthly pregnancy testing. Information on the consequences of pregnancy on the mother and fetus must be discussed.

PHARMACOLOGIC INTERVENTIONS
Calcium Channel Antagonists

Patients who are positive responders to the vasodilator test may be treated with calcium channel blockers.[5] The most commonly used calcium channel blockers are diltiazem, long-acting nifedipine, and amlodipine. Verapamil should be avoided because of its negative inotropic property.[5] Regular follow-up to include functional and hemodynamic reassessment must be performed to determine the need for additional therapies. Patients who do not improve on calcium channel blockers may need alternative or additional therapies.[5]

Diuretics

Diuretics are used to manage right ventricular overload manifested as ascites, lower extremity edema, and elevated jugular venous pressure. Close monitoring of electrolytes and renal function is imperative.[5] Patients must be counseled on a low sodium diet in addition to diuretics.

Anticoagulation

Patients with PAH are at risk for pulmonary embolism from left ventricular compression caused by right ventricular hypertrophy.[5,29] Current guidelines recommend anticoagulation with warfarin in patients with IPAH unless contraindicated, titrated to maintain an international normalized ration of 1.5 to 2.5. Monitoring and follow-up is critical to reduce complications from anticoagulation.[30]

Endothelin Receptor Antagonists

Endothelin-1, a potent vasoconstrictor and proliferative agent is overexpressed in PAH. Two endothelin receptor antagonists are approved in the United States, bosentan (Tracleer, Actelion Pharmaceuticals US, Inc, CA, USA) and ambrisentan (Letairis, Gilead Sciences, Inc, Foster City, CA, USA). Both drugs carry a black box warning on teratogenecity.[5] Pregnancy must be ruled out before drug initiation. Patients of child-bearing age must use 2 forms of contraceptives and take a pregnancy test monthly. The US Food and Drug Administration (FDA) requires that liver function tests be checked monthly for patients on bosentan and hematocrit levels every three months for either drug therapy. There is concern that endothelin antagonists may cause atrophy and male infertility. Counseling is very important before starting these drugs. Because of the risks and safety concerns, these drugs are available through restricted distribution from specialty pharmacies.

Bosentan, a nonselective oral agent is approved for use in functional class II to IV. It has shown to improve 6MW and reduce time to clinical worsening.[37] The starting dose is 62.5 mg twice a day for 4 weeks then increased to 125 mg twice a day.[37] Side effects include potential for hepatotoxicity, anemia, and edema.[37]

Ambrisentan is another oral, once-daily, endothelin A-selective antagonist (ETA)-selective antagonist dosed at 5 or 10 mg.[38] It is approved for functional class II and III symptoms. Side effects include elevation of transaminases, nasal congestion, and lower extremity edema, which occurs more frequently in patients older than 65 years.[38] It is important to differentiate the edema caused by ambrisentan versus edema from disease progression.[5]

Phosphodiesterase Inhibitors

Originally approved for the treatment of erectile dysfunction, phosphodiesterase inhibitors found their place in the treatment of PAH. Vasodilatation occurs by augmenting and sustaining cyclic guanosine 3,5'-monophosphate (cGMP) in the vascular smooth muscle.[5]

Sildenafil (Revatio, Pfizer Labs, NY, USA) is a specific phosphodiesterase 5 inhibitor. Three doses—20 mg, 40 mg, and 80 mg 3 times a day used in clinical trials showed reduction in mean pulmonary artery pressures and improvement in functional class. The incidence of clinical worsening did not differ significantly between the patients treated with sildenafil compared with placebo.[39] The FDA-approved dose is 20 mg 3 times a day. Side effects include headache, epistaxis, flushing, and dyspepsia.[39]

Tadalafil (Adcirca, Lilly, Eli and Company, Indianapolis, IN, USA), a long-acting phosphodiesterase inhibitor, offers a meaningful addition to PAH therapy. The FDA-approved dose of 40 mg, which comes in two 20-mg tablets once daily, improved exercise capacity, clinical worsening, and hemodynamics.[40] The safety profile is similar to that of the lower dose. Headache is the most common side effect.[40]

Prostacyclin

The prostaglandins are potent endogenous vasodilators with antiproliferative properties. Prostanoids have been used for more than 10 years to treat PAH. They act by reducing endothelial cell injury and hypercoagulabiltiy.[30] There are currently 5 commercially available prostanoids: epoprostenol sodium (Flolan, GlaxoSmithKline Pharmaceuticals, NC, USA), epoprostenol for injection (Veletri, Actelion Pharmaceuticals US, Inc, CA, USA), treprostinil sodium (Remodulin, United Therapeutics, MD,

USA), iloprost (Ventavis, Actelion Pharmaceuticals US, Inc, CA, USA), and inhaled treprostinil sodium (Tyvaso, United Therapeutics, MD, USA). The administration and management of these medications is complex and should be limited to facilities with experience and established systematic follow-up.[5] Patients and family must receive extensive education on the disease process as well as medications. In addition, training in the use of appropriate medication inhalation devices or pumps must be accomplished before treatment begins.

Epoprostenol (Flolan) is a potent short-acting vasodilator of the systemic and pulmonary arterial beds.[41] It also inhibits platelet aggregation.[41] The agent has a short half-life and is unstable at room temperature. Its pH value of less than 10.5 requires administration through continuous intravenous infusion with an ice pack. Epoprostenol use in PAH has demonstrated improvement in functional class, hemodynamics, and survival. Side effects include headache, jaw pain, diarrhea, rash, flushing, and arthralgia.[41]

Treprostinil sodium is a synthetic, stable form of prostacyclin with a neutral pH, is stable at room temperature, and has a half-life of 4.5 hours.[42] It can be administered subcutaneously or continuous intravenous infusion. It is FDA approved for functional class II, III, and IV. Treprostinil produced improvement in hemodynamics, exercise tolerance, and signs and symptoms of PAH. Adverse effects of subcutaneous administration include pain or erythema at the site. Other common side effects include headache, nausea, rash, and diarrhea.[42]

Epoprostenol for injection (Veletri) is a synthetic prostaglandin the properties of which are similar to those of epoprostenol sodium (Flolan).[43] It is approved for class III and IV PAH patients. Veletri has a pH of greater than 11, making it room temperature stable at 77°F (25°C). The safety and side effect profile are similar to those of Flolan.[43]

Iloprost is a prostanoid delivered through an aerosol device approved for functional class III and IV PAH. The delivery system produces small particles delivered directly to the alveoli.[44] One disadvantage is its short duration of approximately 1 hour requiring inhalation of 6 to 9 times per day.[44,45] Common side effects include cough, headache, flushing, and jaw pain.[44]

Inhaled treprostinil is a therapy that is added on to improve exercise capacity and quality of life in class III PAH patients who remain symptomatic on bosentan or sildenafil.[46] The dosing interval is 4 hours. The most common adverse events include cough, headache, throat irritation, and nausea.[46]

Although the approved therapies have improved quality of life and outcomes, some patients will decline after their initial treatment because of the progressive nature of PAH.[5] Ongoing follow-up and reassessment of the patients' responses to treatment using prognostic parameters, functional class, exercise endurance, hemodynamic and echocardiographic findings, will guide management to optimize outcomes.[5] The doses of approved PAH medications are in **Table 5**.

INVASIVE THERAPIES

Despite advances in medical therapy for PAH, progressive functional decline caused by worsening right heart failure may occur in certain patients. Surgical interventions, such as atrial septostomy or heart and lung transplantation, may be considered in these patients.[5]

NURSING IMPLICATIONS

Nurses play a critical role in addressing the complex needs of the patients with PH. This role includes educating patients and families about the disease and treatment

Table 5	
Pharmacological options in PAH	
	Dose[a]
Intravenous prostacyclin	
Epoprostenol (Flolan)	Start at 2ng/kg/min
Epoprostenol for injection (Veletri)	Start at 2 ng/kg/min
Treprostinil (Remodulin)	Start at 1.25 ng/kg/min; titrate by 1.25 ng/kg/min per week for the first 4 weeks later 2.5 ng/kg/min per week.
Subcutaneous prostacyclin	
Treprostinil (Remodulin)	Start at 1.25 ng/kg/min; titrate by 1.25 ng/kg/min per week for the first 4 weeks; later 2.5 ng/kg/min per week.
Inhaled prostacyclin	
Iloprost (Ventavis)	Initial dose 2.5 mcg, 6-9 times/day; titrate to 5 mcg, 6-9 times/day, up to 45 mcg per day max. Deliver using the I-neb AAD system
Inhaled treprostinil (Tyvaso)	Initial dose, 3 breaths (18 μg) QID
	Maximum, 9 breaths (54 μg) QID.
	Use with Tyvaso Inhalation System.
Endothelin receptor antagonist	
Bosentan	6.25 mg BID × 4 weeks then increase to 125 mg BID
Ambrisentan	5 or 10 mg daily
Phosphodiesterase inhibitor	
Sildenafil	20 mg TID 4–6 hours apart
Tadalafil	20 mg 2 tablets daily

[a] See full prescribing information.
Abbreviations: BID, twice a day; TID, 3 times a day; QUID, 4 times a day.

options and coordinating the plan of care delivered by a multidisciplinary team. Patients are expected to be partners in the management of their disease. Communication and follow-up should be more frequent in patients with advance symptoms, right heart failure, on parenteral or combination therapy.[5] Additionally, nurses must provide emotional support as well as assistance in navigating the realities associated with having a chronic, incurable disease.

Collaboration with a pulmonary hypertension center is essential to successful patient management. Decision of which therapy to use is complex, requiring joint decision from patient and provider. Identification of potential barriers to care and compliance with medical regimen must be recognized and openly discussed.

Medications to treat PAH are expensive and require safety monitoring. With the exception of phosphodiesterase inhibitors, medications are distributed by specialty pharmacy to ensure that prescribers are familiar with the medication, including required monitoring. Completeness and accuracy of the forms to request medication, including required documents, is vital to avoid delay in therapy. Detailed patient education must be provided to patients and families on medications, importance of regular monthly laboratory monitoring, handling emergent situations, and follow-up. Patients on inhaled, subcutaneous, and intravenous prostacyclin must be trained on mixing their medications and managing inhaled delivery systems, pumps, and cassettes, including trouble shooting. A family member designated as the mixing partner is identified before treatment is initiated. In the event the patient is unable to mix medications, the mixing partner takes over. Patients should have access to their specialty pharmacy and PAH provider at all times. Policies and procedures must be in place addressing treatment of patients who come to the hospital with their own medications and pump. Most hospitals do not stock PAH medications nor have the delivery systems used by patients. Situations such as fractured, clotted, disconnected, or leaking central line; fever; and pump malfunctions may occur, requiring emergent care. The first responders and emergency department staff must have knowledge and training on emergent PAH management to facilitate care and triage of patients. Staff involved in the care of these patients must receive ongoing staff development and training on patient care management and equipment.

SUMMARY

PAH is a chronic disease requiring lifelong therapy, regardless of chosen treatment options. Nurses and other providers must allow for open, honest discussion on the risks and benefits of each therapy. Determining the best treatment option for patients requires consideration of the patient's overall function and social support. These patients benefit from comprehensive and collaborative support from facilities or centers trained in the management of the disease.

REFERENCES

1. Peacock AJ. Treatment of pulmonary hypertension. BMJ 2003;326:835–6.
2. D'Alonzo GE, Barst RJ, Ayres SM, et al. Survival in patients with primary pulmonary hypertension: results from a national prospective registry. Ann Intern Med 1991;115: 343–9.
3. McGoon MD, Torbicki A, Oudiz RJ. Diagnosis and assessment of pulmonary arterial hypertension. In: Barst RJ, editor. Pulmonary arterial hypertension: diagnosis and evidence-based treatment. West Sussex (England): John Wiley and Sons LH; 2008. p. 6–46.
4. Simonneau G, Robbins IM, Beghetti M, et al. Updated clinical classification of pulmonary hypertension. J Am Coll Card 2009;54:S43–54.
5. McLaughlin VV, Archer SL, Badesch DB, et al. ACCF/AHA 2009 Expert consensus document on pulmonary hypertension: a report of the American College of Cardiology Foundation Task Force on Expert Consensus Documents and the American Heart Association developed in collaboration with the American College of Chest Physicians; American Thoracic Society, Inc.; and the Pulmonary Hypertension Association. J Am Coll Cardiol 2009;53:1573–619.
6. Fishman AP. Clinical classification of pulmonary hypertension. Clin Chest Med 2001; 22:385–91.
7. Humbert M, Sitbon O, Chaouat A, et al. Pulmonary arterial hypertension in France: results from a national registry. Am J Respir Crit Care Med 2006;173;1023–30.
8. Rich S, Dantzker DR, Ayres SM, et al. Primary pulmonary hypertension. A national prospective study. Ann Intern Med 1987;107:216–23.
9. Yigla M, Kramer, MR, Bendayan D, et al. Unexplained severe pulmonary hypertension in the elderly: report on 14 patients. Isr Med Assoc J 2004;6:78–81.
10. Cogan JD, Pauciulo MW, Batchman AP, et al. High frequency of BMPR2 exonic deletions/duplications in familial pulmonary arterial hypertension. Am J Respir Crit Care Med 2006;174:590–8.
11. McGoon M, Gutterman D, Steen V, et al. Screening, early detection, and diagnosis of pulmonary arterial hypertension: ACCP evidence-based clinical practice guidelines. Chest 2004;126:14S–34S.

12. Gurtner HP. Aminorex and pulmonary hypertension. A review. Cor Vasa 1985;27(2-3):160–71.

13. Abenhaim L, Moride Y, Brenot F, et al. Appetite -suppressant drugs and the risk of primary pulmonary hypertension. International Primary Pulmonary Hypertension Study Group. N Engl J Med 1996;335:609–16.

14. Gomez-Sanchez MA, Saenz de la Calzada C, Gomez-Pajuelo C, et al. Clinical and pathologic manifestations of pulmonary vascular disease in the toxic oil syndrome. J Am Coll Cardiol 1991;18:1539–45.

15. Sack KE, Criswell LA. Eosinophilia-myalgia syndrome: the aftermath. South Med J 1992;85:878–82.

16. Chin KM, Channick RN, Rubin LJ. Is methamphetamine use associated with idiopathic pulmonary arterial hypertension? Chest 2006;130:16657–63.

17. Hachulla E, Gressin V, Guillevin L, et al. Early detection of pulmonary arterial hypertension in systemic sclerosis: a French nationwide prospective multicenter study. Arthritis Rheum 2005;52:3792–800.

18. Sitbon O, Lascoux-Combe C, Delfraissy JF, et al. Prevalence of HIV-related pulmonary arterial hypertension in the current antiretroviral therapy era. Am J Respir Crit Care Med 2008;177:108–13.

19. Castro M, Krowka MJ, Schroeder DR, et al. Frequency and clinical implications of increased pulmonary artery pressures in liver transplant patients. Mayo Clin Proc 1996;71:543–51.

20. Beghetti M, Galiè N. Eisenmenger syndrome. A clinical perspective in a new era of pulmonary arterial hypertension. J Am Coll Cardiol 2009;53:733–40.

21. Lapa MS, Dias B, Jardim C, et al. Cardio-pulmonary manifestations of hepatosplenic schistosomiasis. Circulation 2009;119:1518–23.

22. Anthi A, Machado RF, Jison ML, et al. Hemodynamic and functional assessment of patients with sickle cell disease and pulmonary hypertension. Am J Respir Crit Care Med 2007;175:1272–9.

23. Gladwin MT, Sachdev V, Jison ML, et al. Pulmonary hypertension as a risk factor for death in patients with sickle cell disease. N Engl J Med 2004;350:886–95.

24. Pietra GG, Capron F, Stewart S, et al. Pathologic assessment of vasculopathies in pulmonary hypertension. J Am Coll Cardiol 2004:43:25S–32S.

25. Cottin V, Nunes H, Brillet PY, et al. Combined pulmonary fibrosis and emphysema: a distinct unrecognized entity. Eur Respir J 2005;26:586–93.

26. Tapson VF, Humbert M. Incidence and prevalence of chronic thromboembolic pulmonary hypertension: from acute to chronic pulmonary embolism. Proc Am Thorac Soc 2006;3:584–8.

27. Jamieson SW, Kapelanski DP, Sakakibara N, et al. Pulmonary endarterectomy: experience and lessons learned in 1,500 cases. Ann Thorac Surg 2003;76:1457–62.

28. Rubin LJ, Hoeper MM, Kleptko W, et al. Current and future management of chronic thromboembolic pulmonary hypertension: from diagnosis to treatment responses. Proc Am Thorac Soc 2006;3:601–7.

29. Gaine SP, Rubin LJ. Primary pulmonary hypertension. Lancet 1998;352:719–25.

30. McLaughlin VV, McGoon MD. Pulmonary arterial hypertension. Circulation 2006;114(13):1417–31.

31. Fedullo PF, Auger WR, Kerr KM, et al. Chronic thromboembolic pulmonary hypertension. N Engl J Med 2001;345:1465–72.

32. Rubin LJ. Diagnosis and management of pulmonary arterial hypertension: ACCP evidence-based clinical practice guidelines. Introduction. Chest 2004;126:7S–10S.

33. Sitbon O, Humbert M, Jais X, et al. Long-term response to calcium channel blockers in idiopathic pulmonary arterial hypertension. Circulation 2005;111:3105–11.

34. Mereles D, Ehlken N, Kreuscher S, et al. Exercise and respiratory training improve exercise capacity and quality of life in patients with severe chronic pulmonary hypertension. Circulation 2006;114:1482–9.

35. Mohr LC. Hypoxia during air travel in adults with pulmonary disease. Am J Med Sci 2008;335:71–9.

36. Weiss BM, Zemp L, Seifert B, et al. Outcome of pulmonary vascular disease in pregnancy: a systematic overview from 1978 through 1996. J Am Coll Cardiol 1998:31:1650–7.

37. Rubin LJ, Badesch DB, Barst RJ, et al. Bosentan therapy for pulmonary arterial hypertension. N Engl J Med 2002;346:896–903.

38. Galiè N, Olschewski H, Oudiz RJ, et al. Ambrisentan for the treatment of pulmonary arterial hypertension: results of the Ambrisentan in Pulmonary Arterial Hypertension, Randomized, Double-Blind, Placebo-Controlled, Multicenter, Efficacy (ARIES) Study 1 and 2. Circulation 2008;117:3010–9.

39. Galiè N, Ghofrani HA, Torbicki A, et al. Sildenafil citrate therapy for pulmonary arterial hypertension. N Engl J Med 2005;353:2148–57.

40. Galiè N, Bundage BH, Ghofrani HA, et al. Tadalafil therapy for pulmonary arterial hypertension. Circulation 2009;119:2894–903.

41. Vane JR, Botting RM. Pharmacodynamic profile of prostacyclin. Am J Cardiol 1995; 75:3A–10A.

42. Tapson VF, Gomberg-Maitland M, McLaughlin VV, et al. Safety and efficacy of IV treprostinil for pulmonary arterial hypertension: a prospective, multicenter, open-label, 12-week trial. Chest 2006;129:683–8.

43. Veletri (epoprostenol for injection) Full Prescribing Information. Actelion Pharmaceuticals US, Inc. 2010. Available at: http://www.veletri.com/patient-prescribing. Accessed January 29, 2011.

44. Gessler T, Schmehl T, Hoeper MM, et al. Ultrasonic versus jet nebulization of iloprost in severe pulmonary hypertension. Eur Respir 2001;17:14–9.

45. Olschewski H, Simmoneau G, Galiè N, et al. Inhaled iloprost for severe pulmonary hypertension. N Engl J Med 2002;347:322–9.

46. McLaughlin VV, Benza RL, Rubin LJ. Addition of inhaled treprostinil to oral therapy for pulmonary arterial hypertension: a randomized controlled clinical trial. J Am Coll Cardiol 2010;58(18):1915–22.

Comprehensive Care of Adults with Acute Ischemic Stroke

Patricia A. Hughes, MSN, RN, CNRN

KEYWORDS

- Stroke • Stroke risk factors • Acute stroke treatment
- Nursing interventions

Stroke is the third leading cause of death in the United States. Approximately 795,000 Americans each year suffer a new or recurrent stroke; 610,000 are first attacks and 185,000 are recurrent attacks.[1,2] Approximately 2.7% of men and 2.5% of women older than the age of 18 had a history of stroke according to data from the 2005 Behavior Risk Factor Surveillance System (BRFSS) Centers for Disease Control and Prevention (CDC).[2] Statistics show that every 40 seconds in the United States, someone suffers a stroke and every 4 minutes someone dies of stroke.[2] Blacks continue to have a higher incidence of stroke, especially among young adults.[1–9] Approximately 40% of stroke deaths occur in males and 60% in females.[10,11] Ischemic strokes account for 87% of strokes and hemorrhagic strokes account for the remaining 13%.[2,4,7,8,11,12] The National Stroke Association now advocates use of the term "brain attack" to reinforce the idea that those exhibiting signs and symptoms of stroke should be treated immediately, as those who experience heart attack should be.[3] Stroke and transient ischemic attacks (TIAs, so-called ministrokes that caused temporary symptoms) account for approximately 1% of emergency department (ED) visits.[13] The purpose of this article is to describe the comprehensive care of adult patients with acute ischemic stroke utilizing the stroke systems of care and the multidisciplinary team approach. Over the past several years, through this system approach and ongoing process improvement, there has been a decrease in stroke mortality and disability.

Stroke remains the leading cause of serious long-term disability in the United States. Direct cost and indirect cost associated with stroke are an estimated $73.7 billion in 2010, according to the American Heart Association. Approximately 55,000 more women than men have a stroke each year.[11] Direct costs are attributed to the initial hospitalization, skilled nursing care, physician and nursing care, medications, durable medical equipment, home health care, and acute rehabilitation. Indirect costs

The author has nothing to disclose.
Baylor University Medical Center, 3500 Gaston Ave., Dallas, TX 75246, USA
E-mail address: pathugh@baylorhealth.edu

Crit Care Nurs Clin N Am 23 (2011) 661–675
doi:10.1016/j.ccell.2011.08.009
0899-5885/11/$ – see front matter © 2011 Elsevier Inc. All rights reserved.

include loss of productivity (loss of future earnings) due to morbidity and mortality and loss of esteem (place in family and society) due to disability.[4,14,15] Mortality rates in the first 30 days after stroke have decreased because of advances in emergency medicine and acute stroke care.[7,8,13,15]

A stroke or "brain attack" occurs when a blood clot blocks an artery or blood vessels breaks, interrupting blood flow to an area of the brain. When either happens brain cells begin to die and brain damage occurs.[5–8,10,11] How a person is affected by the stroke is determined by the location of the stroke and how much of the brain is damaged.[14]

The brain requires 15% to 20% of the total resting cardiac output to provide the necessary glucose and oxygen for its metabolism, despite accounting for only 2% of the body's mass. Seconds after the loss of glucose and oxygen delivery to neurons, the cellular ischemic cascade begins with cessation of the normal electrophysiologic function of the cells. As a result of the neuronal and glial injury, edema occurs in the following hours to days after the stroke, causing injury to the surrounding tissues. Acute treatment in care of the acute ischemic stroke is targeted at preserving the surrounding tissue known as the penumbra.[7,9] The tissue in the penumbra can remain viable for several hours because of marginal tissue perfusion. The cells in the penumbra can be rescued before the irreversible injury occurs by recanalization strategies.

TYPES OF STROKE

There are two types of stroke: ischemic and hemorrhagic. Ischemic stroke accounts for 87% of all strokes.[1,2] Ischemic strokes are caused by reduced or interrupted blood supply to the brain. Without adequate blood flow, tissue death occurs in the region served by the blocked vessel. The most common cause of stroke is thrombosis due to atherosclerosis. Decreased blood flow causes ischemia of brain tissue in the tissue supplied by the affected vessel. The mass of tissue affected may be larger because of the development of considerable edema that compresses the area surrounding the infarct.

Smaller vessel thrombotic stroke (lacunar stroke) typically stems from plaque, diabetes mellitus, or hypertension. The infarct areas are smaller and deficits are less apparent unless it occurs in the internal capsule. Cardioembolic stroke results from atrial fibrillation, valvular heart disease, or ventricular thrombi. Infectious particles, fat, and air or tumor fragments can also cause occlusion of cerebral vessel. Embolism results in blood clots that are easily detached from the wall or valves of the heart and travel to brain. A less common cause of embolism is patent foramen ovale.[5]

Other types of ischemic stroke are caused by prothrombotic states, arterial dissection, arteritis, and drug abuse. For the remaining 30% of ischemic strokes, the etiology is unknown. These strokes are termed cryptogenic.[1]

Hemorrhagic stroke accounts for 13% of strokes. These result from rupture of an artery that causes bleeding onto the surface of the brain (subarachnoid hemorrhage) or into the parenchyma of the brain (intracerebral hemorrhage).[4,6–8,13] Hypertension is the most common cause of hemorrhagic stroke. Rupture of an aneurysm or arteriovenous malformations are less common causes. **Fig. 1** provides a summary of stroke etiologies.

PATHOPHYSIOLOGY OF STROKE

The pathophysiology of stroke can vary depending on the precipitating event. Ischemic–hypoxic brain damage results from decreased cerebral blood flow, either focal or diffuse, which causes hypoxia of cerebral tissue leading to anaerobic

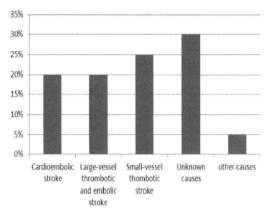

Fig. 1. Etiologies of stroke. (Data from Morrison K. Improving the care of stroke patients. Am Nurse Today 2007;2(4):38–43.)

glycolysis.[6] Decreased blood flow leads to a dense ischemic core surrounded by a marginally perfused area known as the penumbra. A cerebral blood flow (CBF) greater than 25 mL/100 g per minute leads to decreased oxygen and glucose. Cellular swelling and neuronal death follows.

RISKS FACTORS FOR STROKE

Risk factors for stroke can be categorized into two types: modifiable (treatable) and nonmodifiable. Public education should include both risk factor types, with the emphasis being on the modifiable factors that can be controlled by changing lifestyle habits. Evidence shows that management of risk factors leads to significant reductions in the occurrence of both first and recurrent strokes.[1,2,8] Nonmodifiable risk factors are age, gender, race and ethnicity, and family history of cardiovascular disease (**Box 1**). Although stroke is thought of as a disease of the elderly, there has been an increased rate of pediatric stroke in recent years.[2]

CLINICAL PRESENTATION OF STROKE

The clinical manifestation of a stroke is strongly related to which vessel is occluded. If the occlusion occurs in the carotid system, symptoms would be contralateral hemiparesis with facial asymmetry and sensory changes. A homonymous hemianopsoa, Horner's syndrome, amaurosis fugas, or tansmonocular blindess may be seen. Aphasia and headache over ispilateral eye are present if stroke occurs in the left hemisphere lesion. In the right cerebral hemisphere lesion, symptoms include a left visual field deficit, flat affect, constructional apraxic, and dressing apraxia. If the brainstem and cerebellum are affected, hemiparesis or quadriparesis is present, along with face and eye movement abnormalities and diplopia. Oropharyngeal weakness, vertigo, tinnitus, nausea, vomiting, dysmetria, atxia, and dysarthia may also be present.[4,6–9]

STROKE SYSTEMS OF CARE

Many obstacles remained in ensuring that the significant advances and delivery of new effective therapies are translated into clinical practice. These obstacles were related to the fragmentation of stroke care caused by inadequate integration of the various facilities, agencies, and professionals that should closely collaborate in

---

Box 1
Stroke risk factors[4–8,12,14–16]

Nonmodifiable Risk Factors

Gender

Race/ethnicity

Family history of CVA

Family history of cardiovascular disease

Modifiable Risk Factors

Hypertension

Diabetes mellitus

Smoking

Alcohol intake

Sedentary lifestyle

Obesity

Atrial fibrillation

Drug abuse

Less Common Risk Factors

Metabolic syndrome

---

providing stroke care.[17] The American Heart Association and American Stroke Association (AHA/ASA) created a task force to define the key components and methods for encouraging the implantation of a stroke system of care.

The goal of every hospital seeking or that has obtained certification as a primary stroke center is to provide the best possible outcome for patients suffering a stroke.[18] An organized, evidence-based approach to each aspect of stroke care contributes to the quality of the outcomes and requires an infrastructure that the organized center can provide.[17] Coordinated care of the acute ischemic stroke patient results in improved outcomes, decreased lenght of stay, and decreased costs.[6,12]

In 2000, the Brain Attack Coalition proposed the creation of two types of stroke centers: the Primary Stroke Center (PSC) and the Comprehensive Stroke Center (CSC). The concept was born after experts in the field realized that fewer than 5% of people with an acute stroke received tissue plasminogen activator (rtPA), a medication that when given within 3 hours of the beginning of stroke symptoms can help dissolve stroke-causing blood clots. However, if given later, it can lead to serious bleeding in the brain.[7,8,17,19,20]

The ASA task force developed reommendations on the organization and operation of systems of care for the treatment of stroke patients throughout the United States, including both ischemic and hemorrhagic subtypes.[8,15,18,21] Stroke systems of care should be able to provide key aspects of stroke care. Those key elements include acute stroke intervention and management, prevention of complications, secondary stroke prevention, and early rehabilitation.

The Brain Attack Coalition set forth recommendations for facilities to become certified as a Primary Stroke Center. **Box 2** lists the requirements for primary stroke center.

Box 2
Criteria for primary stroke center certification[4,6–9,12,15,16,21,22]

1. A CT scan or MRI scanner must be available 24 hours each day, and should be reserved for stroke patients within 25 minutes of being ordered

2. Access to neurosurgical services (access to a brain surgeon) must be provided.

3. Laboratory tests of patients with acute stroke must be completed within 45 minutes of being ordered.

4. A physician with expertise in interpreting CT or MRI studies must be available within 20 minutes of being asked to read a study.

5. A written t-PA protocol must exist in the ED.

6. The medical organization must have a declared and established commitment for acute stroke care.

7. The hospital must have written acute stroke "clinical pathways" or "care maps."

8. An acute stroke team, including a physician and at least one other health care professional, must be available around the clock.

9. Follow long-term stroke treatment outcomes, and design quality improvement activities.

10. Emergency staff must have completed formal training in acute stroke treatments.

11. The hospital must have a "stroke unit."

12. There must be a designated stroke center director.

13. The stroke team must schedule stroke medical education sessions for stroke staff.

14. The hospital must provide formal stroke training for ambulance personnel.

A Comprehensive Stroke Center not only meets the requirements for a primary stroke center but also has the capabilities to provide interventional neuroradiologists as part of a stroke team. The neuroradiologists are available 24 hours a day, 7 days a week to mobilize quickly and utilize the advanced intra-arterial and mechanical embolectomy techniques.[8] The Joint Commission (TJC) currently offers Primary Stroke Center Certification. It is anticipated that in the future certification will be offered for a more complex level of stroke care.

In 2007, the ASA published a scientific statement published in *Stroke*, Guidelines for the Early Management of Adults with Ischemic Stroke.[8] This was an update to the initial guidelines published in 2003. The current guideline provides the classes and levels of evidence used in recommendations for care of patients with stroke.

STROKE CARE

Acute ischemic stroke is a medical emergency and will always be time dependent, with the best outcomes resulting from the earliest intervention.[6,8,9] Stroke management is a team effort, with the nursing and medical staff working closely together.[4,6,8,14]

Pre-hospital Stroke Care

The emergency medical services play a key role in the success of acute stroke intervention. Upon responding, they can obtain important information about the time of onset and perform a quick neurologic assessment, and can identify patients who may be candidates for interventional therapy.[8,9] Emergency medical services (EMS)

Table 1 Stroke evaluation time benchmarks[4,6–8,15,17,18,20]	
Time Interval	**Target Time**
Door to doctor	10 minutes
Access to neurologic expertise	15 minutes
Door to CT scan completion	25 minutes
Door to CT scan interpretation	45 minutes
Door to drug/treatment	60 minutes
Admission to monitored bed	3 hours

From recommendations by the NINDS and ACLS.

personnel should be trained to administer validated pre-hospital quick neurologic assessment such as the Cincinnati Pre-hospital Stroke Scale (CPSS) that tests arm strength, facial symmetry, and speech. The CPSS and the Los Angeles Pre-hospital Stroke Screen (LAPSS) have been widely accepted among pre-hospital personnel and physicians as an effective means to identify stroke victims who may be candidates for interventional therapy. Education for emergency medical service personnel now includes stroke education for this purpose.[8,9,18] Pre-hospital notification of the arrival of the patient to the ED expedites evaluation and diagnosis.[7–9,15]

Stroke experts have developed in-hospital time intervals to allow stroke patients to be treated and evaluated in an expedient manner. Advance Cardiac Life Support (ACLS) and the National Institute of Neurological Disorders and Stroke (NINDS) have set forth stroke evaluation time benchmarks for potential thrombolytic candidates, summarized in **Table 1**.

Acute Phase: Thrombolytic Therapy in Acute Ischemic Stroke

Restoring blood flow in the affected artery is the primary aim of treatment in the acute phase of acute ischemic stroke and is a predictor of outcome. Intravenous rtPA remains the only U.S. Food and Drug Administration (FDA) approved thrombolytic agent for acute ischemic stroke within 3 hours of symptom onset. Success of recanalization therapy depends on timing as well as degree of reperfusion. Various pharmaceutical agents and devices, used alone as well as in combination, have been used to achieve recanalization in acute ischemic stroke.[7,8,18,19]

In a 1995 NINDS trial, patients given rtPA had a significant reduction in disability at 30 days, with no difference in mortality.[8,18] By 30 days, 43% of those enrolled were functionally independent. At 3 months, 50% of those treated had minimal or no disability versus 38% of controls. Further, at 3 months, significantly more patients given rtPA had minimal or no disability when compared to those given a placebo. By 90 days, 11% to 13% more of those treated with rtPA had significant improvements in functionality and reduced disability. One of every 11 stroke patients treated in an ED with rtPA will leave the hospital with little or no disability.[8,19,20] These results were recently substantiated by a larger trial (Standard Treatment with Alteplase to Reverse Stroke. [STARS] Study) involving 57 hospitals.[2] Thrombolytic therapy for acute ischemic stroke is endorsed by the American Academy of Neurologists and the AHA. In severe stroke (NINDS scores >20), the chance of an elderly person having complete recovery increases from 0% to 7% to 8% with rtPA.[8,19,20] This offsets the 3% increased risk of death, and the increased risk of symptomatic intracranial hemorrhage, associated with the drug.[7,8,19]

The evidence supporting the use of thrombolytic therapy in stroke includes 21 completed randomized controlled clinical trials enrolling 7152 patients, using various agents, doses, time windows, and intravenous or intra-arterial modes of administration.[8,19,20] Determination of the time of onset of symptoms is critical in deciding eligibility for thrombolytic therapy. On-label treatment must be initiated within 3 hours of onset of symptoms. Sometimes the precise onset time cannot be determined with certainty. For example, when a patient awakens with a deficit after a night's sleep or after a nap or is found stricken and unable to communicate the onset time. In these instances, the onset time is taken as the last time the patient was known to be well. Caution should be exercised in patients with neglect syndromes who may not have observed their onset time reliably.[4,7,8,19]

In 2009, the AHA/ASA published guidelines that expanded the time window for treatment of acute ischemic stroke with intravenous rtPA to a 3- to 4.5-hour window based on prospective study by the European Cooperative Acute Stroke Study (ECASS)-3.[8,9,19,20] The ECASS-3 trial represents an important advancement in the treatment of acute ischemic stroke. The results are consistent with previous studies and pooled analyses of previous trials in this time window, providing level B evidence. Intravenous rtPA can be given safely to carefully selected patients within 3 to 4.5 hours after stroke. When given in this time period, rtPA can improve outcomes after stroke in a selected group of patients.[7,8,19,20] The AHA/ASA continues to advocate for early treatment, stating that although a longer time window for treatment has been tested formally, delays in evaluation and initiation of therapy should be avoided, because the opportunity for improvement is greater with earlier treatment.

Stroke patient triage and care on arrival to the ED is considered a level two of a five-level emergency severity index system. A level two index means in need of immediate assessment category. Included in this category is unstable trauma or critical care cardiac patients. ED nurses and all other staff must know the NINDS benchmark treatment time for acute ischemic stroke is 60 minutes of arrival in the ED.[13]

In the ED, the priorities are to stabilize the patient, take a complete history, and obtain a computed tomography (CT) scan, which is critical in determining whether the stroke is an infarction or intracerebral hemorrhage and to exclude nonvascular lesions.[13] According to the scientific statement by the AHA, early implementation of stroke pathways and stroke team notification should occur in parallel with the ED evaluation and management.[7–9,13,19]

Immediate evaluation of suspected stroke includes stabilization of the ABCs (airway, breathing, circulation), neurologic deficits, and possible comorbidities. The overall goal is to exclude stroke mimics and identify other conditions requiring immediate intervention. This permits determination of potential causes of the stroke for early secondary prevention.[7–9,19]

When conducting the medical history, the last known time the patient felt well is the most important piece of information needed to determine the course of treatment for the patient suspected of acute ischemic stroke.[4,7–9,16,19] For the physician, the last known time the patient was seen normal is crucial in assessing the patients eligibility for thrombolytic therapy. Family members or friends are a crucial part of care and providing this information. Any comorbid conditions should be ascertained. A history of diabetes, hypertension, seizures, trauma, myocardial infarction, cardiac arrhythmias such as atrial fibrillation, or history of prior stroke or TIA and what medications patient is currently taking will be crucial in the prethrombolytic assessment phase. The health care provider especially needs to know if patient is currently receiving anticoagulation therapy. It is extremely important during the workup phase to rule out stroke mimics that can present in postseizure patients.

Thrombolytic therapy should be implemented only when a physician with expertise in stroke establishes a diagnosis of ischemic stroke, and a physician with appropriate expertise in reading CT is available.[8,19] The clinical diagnosis of ischemic stroke should include a measurable neurologic deficit and should be based on an acceptable stroke-severity scale such as the National Institute of Health Stroke Scale (NIHSS). A prethrombolytic assessment is required for all potential candidates for thrombolytic therapy (**Box 3**).

IV Administration of Thrombolytic Therapy

A blood pressure greater than 185 mm Hg systolic and diastolic greater than 110 mm Hg is a contraindication to intravenous rtPA. The rtPA dose for acute ischemic stroke is less than the recommended dose for myocardial infarction or pulmonary embolism. When prepared, there is 100 mg of the drug in the vial. Dosing is weight based, with the total dose not to exceed 90 mg. The remaining portion of the preparation should be discarded to prevent accidental overdose. The dose must be reconstituted by a pharmacist, or in some institutions, by the nurse administering the medication. It must verified by a second licensed staff member (pharmacist, nurse, or physician) after reconstitution, before administration. Nurses should be educated in reconstitution of rtPa. The drug is administered as follows: 10% of the drug is given as a bolus intravenously over 1 minute, and the remaining 90% is administered as a continuous infusion over the next 60 minutes.

Nursing care of patients receiving intravenous rtPA is shown in **Table 2**, and includes frequency of vital signs and neurologic assessment. An additional nursing intervention for consideration includes insertion of Foley catheter. The Foley catheter should be placed before thrombolytic therapy if there are any questions about mobility afterwards. Nasogastric tubes or central lines should be inserted for 24 hours if not placed before treatment with intravenous rtPA.

Anticoagulants/antiplatelet agents are not to be given for 24 hours after administering rtPA. Blood laboratory work monitored includes a complete blood count, prothromin time, partial prothrombin time, international normalized ratio (INR), and fibrinogen. Patients should also have a NIHSS assessment every twelve hours for the first 24 hours after thrombolytic therapy.

Blood Glucose Control

Hyperglycemia has been show to be associated with a poor outcome and reduced reperfusion in thrombolytic as well as extension of the infarcted territory. Blood sugar should be tightly maintained within goal range (90–140 mg/dL).[4,6–9,19] Patients who have normal blood glucose should not be given intravenous fluids containing excessive glucose, which could lead to hyperglycemia and may exacerbate ischemic injury.[4,6–9,19] Studies have shown that an elevated serum glucose is common in the acute phase of stroke and may be related to uncontrolled or undetected diabetes mellitus or stress-induced hyperglycemia associated with cortisol and norepinephrine release at the time of the insult.[4,8,9] Hyperglycemia has been attributed to increased length of stay and increased mortality at 30 days, as well as increased costs.[4,8] An insulin protocol should be used to maintain blood glucose less than 140 mg/dL.[4,6–8,16] Nurses should follow individual hospital policies and procedures.

Box 3
Prethrombolytic assessment checklist[2,4,6,8,9,16,18,19,21]

Indications for Treatment

Acute ischemic stroke symptoms

Symptoms onset within 3 hours of treatment

CT of head without intracranial hemorrhage or pathology other than acute ischemic stroke

Age >18 years

Contraindications to Treatment

SBP >185 or DBP >110 mm Hg despite treatment

Seizure at onset

Recent surgery/trauma (<15 days)

Recent intracranial or spinal surgery, head trauma, or stroke (<3 months)

History of ICH, brain aneurysm, or vascular malformation or brain tumor

Active internal bleeding (<22 days)

Platelets <100,000, PTT >40 seconds after heparin use, or PT >15, or INR >1.7, or known bleeding diathesis

Suspicion of subarachnoid hemorrhage

CT findings (ICH, SAH, or major infarct signs)

Pregnancy

Additional Contraindications for Patients Treated Between 3 and 4.5 Hours

Patient >80 years old

Any anticoagulant use prior to admission (even if INR <1.7)

NIHSS >25

Prior history of *both* stroke and diabetes

CT findings of >1/3 middle cerebral artery (MCA) territory

Relative contraindications:

  1. Advanced age

  2. Glucose <50 or >400

  3. Life expectancy <1 year or severe comorbid illness or CMO on admission

  4. Rapid improvement or stroke severity too mild

  5. Care team unable to determine eligibility

  6. Increased risk of bleeding due to comorbid conditions

  7. Pt/family refused

  8. Stroke severity NIHSS >22

Blood Pressure Management

Maintenance of perfusion to the ischemic area is the goal of blood pressure control. Studies have shown aggressive lowering of blood pressure can cause neurologic worsening; therefore a reasonable goal would be to lower blood pressure by 15% to 25% within the first day.[8,9] A decline in blood pressure occurs within the first hours

Table 2
Nursing care of patients with acute ischemic stroke

Schedule of neurologic assessment and vital signs and other acute care assessments in thrombolysis-treated and nonthrombolysis–treated patients

Thrombolysis-Treated Patients	Nonthrombolysis–Treated Patients
Neurologic assessment and vital signs (except temperature) every 15 minutes during rtPA infusion, then every 30 minutes for 6 hours, then every 60 minutes for 16 hours (total of 24 hours). Note: Frequency of BP assessments may need to be increased if systolic BP stays ≥180 mm Hg or diastolic BP stays ≥105 mm Hg. Temperature reading every 4 hours or as required. Treat temperatures >99.6°F with acetaminophen as ordered.	In ICU, every hour with neurological checks or more frequently if necessary. In non-ICU setting, depending on patient's condition and neurological assessments, at a minimum check neurological assessment and vital signs every 4 h
Call physician if systolic BP >185 or <110 mm Hg; diastolic BP >105 or <60 mm Hg; pulse <50 or >110 beats per minute; respirations >24 per minute; temperature >99.6°F; or for worsening of stroke symptoms or other decline in neurologic status.	Call physician for further treatment based on physician and institutional preferences/guidelines: Systolic BP >220 or <110 mm Hg; diastolic BP >120 or <60 mm Hg; pulse <50 or >110 per min; temperature >99.6°F; respirations >24 per min; or for worsening of stroke symptoms or other decline in neurological status
For O$_2$ saturation <92%, give O$_2$ by cannula at 2–3 L/min.	For O$_2$ saturation <92%, give O$_2$ by cannula at 2–3 L/min
Monitor for major and minor bleeding complications.	N/A
Continuous cardiac monitoring up to 72 hours or more.	Continuous cardiac monitoring for 24–48 hours
Measure intake and output.	Measure intake and output
Provide bed rest.	Bed rest
IV fluids NS at 75–100 mL/h.	IV fluids NS at 75–100 mL/h
No heparin, warfarin, aspirin, clopidogrel, or dipyridamole for 24 hours, then start antithrombotic as ordered.	Antithrombotics should be ordered within first 24 h of hospital admission
Brain CT or MRI after rtPA therapy.	Repeat brain CT scan or MRI may be ordered 24 to 48 h after stroke or as needed

BP, blood pressure; ICU, intensive care unit; IV, intravenous; MRI, magnetic resonance imaging; N/A, not applicable; NS, normal saline.
From Summers D, Leonard A, Wentworth D, et al. Comprehensive overview of nursing and interdisciplinary care of the acute ischemic stroke patient: a scientific statement from the American Heart Association. Stroke 2009;40:2911–44; with permission of American Heart Association.

after stroke even without any specific medical treatment in a majority of patients.[8,23] AHA guidelines recommend that blood pressure should not be treated in the hyperacute period unless the systolic blood pressure is greater than 220 mm Hg or diastolic blood pressure is greater than 120 mm Hg with repeated measurements.[8]

The first drug of choice for lowering blood pressure is {labetalol 10 to 20 mg IV over 1 to 2} minutes and may be repeated one time. If the blood pressure goal is not achieved, nitroglycerine paste 1 to 2 inches should be applied. {Nicardipine infusion may be initiated at 5 mg/h.} The infusion can be titrated up by 2.5 mg per hour at 5- to 15-minute intervals with a maximum infusion rate of 15 mg per hour.[8,9]

Anticoagulants

The goals of anticoagulant therapy are to prevent early recurrent embolus, assist in maintaining collateral blood flow, and halt progression of a thrombus.[5] Warfarin is the most common oral anticoagulant used mainly in cardioembolic stroke. The internationalized normalized ratio (INR) is usually monitored with a desired range of 2 to 2.5. Antiplatelet therapy should be initiated in the absence of acute bleeding after the first 24 hours after the administration of rtPA.

Temperature Management

Evidence has shown that fever appears to exacerbate the ischemic injury to neurons and is associated with increased morbidity and mortality in acute stroke.[4,8] Increased metabolic demands and free radical production are cited as the cause for this additional injury. Maintaining normal temperature improves the outcome in stroke patients.[4,6–9] Recommendations by the Stroke Study Group are to begin acetaminophen when the temperature is at 99.6°F or higher.[8] Other cooling methods such as hypothermia cooling machines can be used to maintain normal temperature.

Studies have shown patients suffering acute ischemic stroke have better outcomes if cared for in designated stroke units.[4,8,21] Nurses who work in the stroke unit nurses are specially educated to care for stroke patients. The care of patients in the stroke unit is guided by clinical pathways and protocols that are required for primary stroke centers (see **Table 2**). Nurse-to-patient ratios in the acute stroke unit and the intensive care unit are generally lower than on a general floor because of the complexity of a newly diagnosed stroke patient. If the patient has received intravenous or intra-arterial rtPA the nurse must monitor for bleeding, which is a major complication of the medication. Frequent neurologic assessments should be made to monitor for any deterioration in the patient's condition and for early signs of bleeding. This is crucial in the early phase of stroke and throughout the patient's hospital stay. The NIHSS provides valuable information on the severity of the stroke, trends progress of the patient's neurologic status, and can be used as an effective tool in the discharge planning process. The patient needs to be continuously monitored for aspiration pneumonia and seizures. Nursing staff should be aware of the signs and symptoms of cerebral edema, hemorrhage, and angioedema.

All patients with acute ischemic stroke should be assessed for dysphagia before oral intake and receive physical, occupational, and speech therapy evaluation on arrival to the stroke unit. Nursing interventions include assessment of the patient's respiratory status and the patient's ability to clear secretions. Oxygen saturation should be maintained greater than 92%.[4,6] The head of the bed should be elevated at least 30°. These patients are at risk of aspiration and development of cerebral edema. Studies have shown that elevation head of the bed maximizes oxygenation and increases blood flow to the brain.[6] A nasogastric tube should be placed for administration of medications and for nutritional needs for patients who are unable to swallow. Tube feedings are started based on dietitian recommendations. It is necessary to wait for 24 hours to insert a nasogastric tube for the patient who received rtPA, if not placed before receiving the thrombolytic. Care Coordination and Social Work should begin the discharge planning process on arrival. The nurse serves as the patient advocate and is instrumental in coordinating the care of the patient on a daily basis (see **Table 2**).

Acute Stroke Interventions

Intra-arterial (IA) infusion of thrombolytic agents within 6 hours of symptom onset has been shown to be effective in reestablishing flow in cerebral artery occlusions with improved clinical outcomes. Combining intravenous therapy with intra-arterial rtPA has been shown to be as safe and effective as intravenous therapy in a nonrandomized trial. One obstacle is the relatively small number of hospitals offering this option.[8,9,18]

There are other available options for treatment in the 6- to 8-hour window after stroke symptoms occur such as mechanical embolectomy. The first device, the Merci Retriever, was approved in 2007 by the FDA for removal of clots from intracerebral arteries. The device utilizes a tiny flexible wire that is inserted from the groin up through the blocked artery, where the coiled wire is deployed. The coil grabs the clot and pulls it into the catheter. The Merci Retriever can be used in combination with rtPa. Expanding the treatment window from 3 hours for intravenous rtPa to 6 to 8 hours with intra-arterial thrombolysis or mechanical embolectomy could dramatically increase the number of patients with acute ischemic stroke who are eligible for treatment.[18] In 2008, the Penumbra system became available for use. This system helps restore brain flow by using suction to grab clots in the brain for treatment of acute embolic stroke. The device is safe to use up to 8 hours after stroke.[7–9,18,20,22]

CERTIFIED PRIMARY STROKE CENTERS

To maintain certification as a primary stroke center, hospitals must demonstrate adherence to evidence-based care of patients hospitalized with stroke. Get with the Guidelines-Stroke (GTWG) is the AHA/ASA collaborative performance improvement program. The GWTG–Stroke development began in 2001, modeling the GWTG program for acute myocardial infarction. In 2003 the GTWG–Stroke program was tested to determine if it could provide hospitals with the tools needed to improve care for stroke patients. In April 2004, the GTWG–Stroke was made available to all hospitals in the United States.[23] Stroke measures apply to processes and aspects of care that are strongly supported by science. The GTWG–Stroke allows for PSCs to measure and evaluate treatment and track facility adherence to the guidelines, both individually and against national benchmarks over time.

In 2010, stroke became a national hospital core measure, derived from a set of quality indicators defined by the Centers for Medicare and Medicaid Services (CMS). Core measures have been shown to reduce the risk of complications, prevent recurrences, and otherwise treat the majority of patients who come to a hospital for treatment of a condition or illness. These help improve the quality of patient care by focusing on the actual results of care. CMS publicly reports data relating to the core measures. The eight core measures for stroke are listed in **Box 4**.

SUMMARY

Stroke continues to represent the leading cause of long term disability despite positive achievements in the last few years. An estimated 50 million stroke survivors world wide currently cope with significant physical, cognitive, and emotional deficits, and 25% to 74% of these survivors will require some assistance or are fully dependent on caregivers for activities of daily living.[14]

Box 4
Stroke core measures

STK-1: Venous thromboembolism (VTE) prophylaxis: Ischemic and hemorrhagic stroke patients who received VTE prophylaxis or have documentation why no VTE prophylaxis was given the day or the day after hospital admission.

STK-2: Discharged on antithrombotic therapy: Ischemic stroke patient's prescribed antithrombotic therapy at hospital discharge.

STK-3: Anticoagulation therapy for atrial fibrillation/flutter: Ischemic stroke patients with atrial fibrillation/flutter who are prescribed anticoagulation therapy at hospital discharge.

STK-4: Thrombolytic therapy: Acute ischemic stroke patients who arrive at this hospital within 2 hours of time last known well and for whom IV t-PA was initiated at this hospital within 3 hours of time last know well.

STK-5: Antithrombotic therapy by end of hospital day 2: Ischemic stroke patients administered antithrombotic therapy by the end of hospital day 2.

STK-6: Discharged on statin medication: Ischemic stroke patients with LDL ≥100 mg/dL, or LDL not measured, or who were on a lipid-lowering medication before hospital arrival are prescribed statin medication at hospital discharge.

STK-8: Stroke education: Ischemic or hemorrhagic stroke patients or their caregivers who were given educational materials during the hospital stay addressing all of the following: activation of emergency medical system, need for follow-up after discharge, medications prescribed at discharge, risk factors for stroke, and warning signs and symptoms of stroke.

STK-10: Assess for rehabilitation: Ischemic or hemorrhagic stroke patients who were assessed for rehabilitation services.

STK-7: Dysphagia screening and STK 9: smoking cessation were retired effective Jan. 2010.

Based on measure information from the Specifications Manual for National Hospital Inpatient Quality Measures Version 3.2.

The interdisciplinary team approach, with the nurse playing the central role, is important across the continuum of care. Families must cope with the impact of stoke on their daily lives once the acute phase of stroke care is over. Studies have shown personal and environmental factors influence outcomes after stroke.[14] Patient and family education during the acute phase of stroke care is vitally important. There is also a need to educate nursing and other members of the interdisciplinary team about the potential for recovery in the later or more chronic phases of stroke care.[6]

The goal of hospitals seeking and obtaining certification as a Primary Stroke Center is to provide the best possible outcomes for patients suffering a stroke. An organized evidence-based approach to each aspect of stroke care contributes to the quality of the outcomes and requires an infrastructure that the organized center can provide.[18]

Stroke is a complex disease process that requires the skills of an interdisciplinary team.[4] Prevention of medical complications and neurologic deterioration is key in managing patients with acute ischemic stroke. The use of clinical pathways and physician standing orders helps to guide the team in managing the care of stroke patients in the acute phase of care.[4] Traditionally the role of educating patients and families about the modifiable and treatable risk factors, and the nonmodifiable risk factors for stroke has been a nursing responsibility. Because patient education is a performance standard for primary stroke centers, nurses must be well informed regarding evidence-based practices associated with effective lifestyle modification strategies for a diverse population.[4,6,14]

REFERENCES

1. National Center of Health Statistics. Available at: www.cdc.gov/nchs/hci:htm. Accessed April 9, 2011.
2. Ver'ronique R, Go Al D, Donald, et al. Heart disease and stroke statistics 2011. Circulation 2011;123:e65–e83. Available at: http://circ.ahajournals.org. Accessed September 4, 2011.
3. Sauerbeck L. Primary stroke prevention. AJN 2006;106(11):40–5.
4. Summers D, Leonard A, Wentworth D, et al. Comprehensive overview of nursing and interdisciplinary care of the acute ischemic stroke patient: a scientific statement from the American Heart Association. Stroke 2009;40:2911–44.
5. Chulay M, Burns S. AACN essentials of critical care nursing. 2nd edition. New York: McGraw-Hill; 2010. p. 307–11.
6. Bader M, Littlejohns L. AANN core curriculum for neuroscience nursing. 4th edition. St. Louis (MO): Elsevier; 2004.
7. Sharma M, Clark H, Armour T. Acute stroke: evaluation and treatment. Agency for Healthcare Research and Quality, U.S. Department of Health & Human Services. Available at: www.ahrq.gov/clinic/epcsums/acstrokesum.htm. Accessed April 8, 2008.
8. Adams H, del Zoppo G, Alberts M. Guidelines for the early management of adults with ischemic stroke. Stroke 2007;38:1655–711.
9. Jauch E, Kissela, B. Acute stroke management. Available at: http://emedicine, medscape.com/article/1159752. Accessed January 21, 2011.
10. National Stroke Association. Stroke fact sheet, November 2009.
11. National Stroke Association. Stroke 101. Available at: www.stroke.org. Accessed January 21, 2011.
12. Morrison K. Improving the care of stroke patients. Am Nurse Today 2007;2(4):38–43.
13. Kellicker P, Schub T. Stroke treatment strategies in the emergency department. Cinahal Information Systems, June, 2010.
14. Miller E, Murray L, Richards L, et al. Comprehensive overview of nursing and interdisciplinary rehabilitation care of the stroke patient. Stroke 2010; 41. Available at: http://stroke.ahajournals.org. Accessed January 21, 2011.
15. Schamm L, Fayad P, Acker J, et al. Translating evidence into practice: a decade of efforts by the American Heart Association/American Stroke Association to reduce death and disability due to stroke. Stroke 2010;41:1051–65. Available at: http://stroke.ahajournals.org/cgi/content/full/41/5/1051. Accessed January 21, 2011.
16. Goldstein L, Bushnell C, Adams R, et al. 2010 Guidelines for the primary prevention of stroke. Stroke 2010;42:517–84.
17. Schwamm L, Pancioli A, Acker J. Recommendations for the establishment of stroke systems of care. Stroke 2005;36:1–9.
18. Rymer M, Thrutchley D. Organizing regional networks to increase acute stroke intervention. Neurol Res 2005;27.
19. Saver J, Kalafut M. Thrombolytic therapy in stroke. Available at: Emedicine. medscape.com. Accessed January 21, 2011.
20. Del Zoppo G, Saver J, Jauch E. Expansion for the time window for treatment of acute ischemic stroke with intravenous tissue plasminogen activator: a science advisory from the American Heart Association/American Stroke Association. Stroke 2009;40; 294–8. Available at: http://stroke.ahajournals.org/cgi/content/full/40/8/2945. Accessed January 21, 2011.

21. Vega J. Primary stroke centers provide superior care for stroke patients. Available at: http://stroke.about.com/od/caregiverresources/a/StrokeUnit.htm. Accessed January 15, 2011.
22. Rhmer M. Building a stroke center: a systems approach to better outcomes. Endovasc Today May, 2007;52-7.
23. Phillips SJ. Pathophysiology and management of hypertension in acute ischemic stroke. Hypertension 1994;23:131–6.

Diabetes and Cardiovascular Disease

Barbara Leeper, MN, RN-BC, CNS M-S, CCRN

KEYWORDS

• Diabetes • Glucose management • Critical care
• Cardiovascular disease

Diabetes is increasing at a rapid rate in the United States. The prevalence of diabetes for all age groups is estimated to be approximately 23.6 million individuals, representing 7.8% of the population. There are 1.6 million new cases diagnosed every year, which can be attributed to the increasing incidence of type 2 diabetes. Nearly 18 million individuals have been diagnosed with diabetes while 5.7 million remain undiagnosed. Experts estimate an additional 57 million Americans are at high risk for diabetes.[1] Thirty-eight percent of patients admitted to the hospital are diabetics. It is estimated that 26% have been diagnosed while the remaining 12% have no history of diabetes. Current evidence links hyperglycemia in hospitalized patients to poorer outcomes. Further, mortality rates are higher in newly diagnosed diabetics.[2,3]

The cost of hyperglycemia is significant, with a 2002 estimate of $132 billion in the United States. Direct care costs accounted for $92 billion while $40 billion was attributed to indirect costs including time lost from work and disability.[4] Krinsley and Jones conducted an economic analysis of 1600 patients before and after intensive glycemic management.[5] Findings demonstrated a cost reduction during the treatment period in the amount of $1,339,500 or $1580 per patient.[5] Ventilator hours decreased by 34.3%, and intensive care unit (ICU) length of stay (days) decreased by 13.9%, with a projected cost savings of approximately $800,000 for these two measures.[5]

Van den Berghe and colleagues conducted a post hoc analysis on data from a previous large randomized controlled trial conducted in a surgical ICU. These results also showed significant cost reductions in patients who were in the intensive insulin treatment group, demonstrating the benefits of glucose control in critically ill patients in the ICU.[6]

The purpose of this article is to discuss issues related to glucose control in the cardiovascular and critical care patient populations, supporting the case for better glycemic management in hospitalized cardiovascular and critically ill patients with

The author has nothing to disclose.
Cardiovascular Services, Baylor University Medical Center, 3500 Gaston Avenue, Dallas, TX 75246, USA
E-mail address: Bobbi.Leeper@baylorhealth.edu

diabetes. Problems associated with blood glucose variability and blood glucose measurements are presented, followed by a discussion of nursing practice issues.

DIABETES AND CARDIOVASCULAR DISEASE

Diabetes is a known risk factor for cardiovascular disease (CVD). Individuals with type 1 and type 2 diabetes are 4 to 10 times more likely to develop CVD than nondiabetic individuals.[7] The atherosclerotic process has been found to be more advanced in diabetic individuals, evidenced by carotid intima–media thickness measures or coronary calcium scores.[7] The pathophysiology of accelerated atherosclerosis and development of CVD in the diabetic is complex. Type 1 diabetic patients are often diagnosed at a young age, with many years passing between the onset of diabetes mellitus (DM) and the diagnosis of CVD. The exact cause of the accelerated atherosclerotic process is unknown. Some believe the onset of CVD in the type 1 patient with DM can be attributed to "weight gain" or abdominal adiposity resulting from years of hyperinsulinemia. The abdominal fat may contribute to insulin resistance and the pro-atherogenic process similar to what occurs in the individual with Type 2 DM. Others believe the CVD is due to the adverse effects of diabetic microangiopathy.[7]

Patients with type 2 diabetes usually have hypertension. A number of abnormalities exist in systemic lipoprotein metabolism, inflammatory and coagulation pathways that are known to be proatherogenic. These are related to the coexisting insulin resistance in many type 2 diabetic patients. The result is increased levels of low-density lipoproteins, triglycerides, postprandial lipemia, and elevated levels of C-reactive protein, plasminogen activator 1, and fibrinogen. As a result, there is an increased risk for CVD. Insulin resistance in type 2 patients with DM is thought to be related to abdominal adiposity and accumulation of fat in the visceral fat depot.[7]

In spite of controlling blood pressure and use of statin-type medications for reducing cholesterol levels, there continues to be a residual incremental risk for the development of CVD in patients with diabetes. A particular challenge is the increasing rates of diabetes in developed countries that is associated with improved nutrition and increased obesity. Some suggest the incidence of diabetes in the United States will nearly double within the next two to three decades.[7] In addition, younger patients are being diagnosed with Type 2 diabetes, making them more vulnerable to CVD at a younger age.[7]

GLUCOSE CONTROL IN CARDIAC SURGERY PATIENTS

It is well known that patients who are diabetic are at increased risk for infections after major surgery.[8] It is believed that several factors contribute to this risk, particularly the impairment of the immune response, especially the neutrophils. In patients with diabetes, neutrophils have been found to have impaired chemotaxis, oxidative burst, and phagocytosis. Some believe hyperglycemia appears to contribute to this impaired neutrophil reactivity. One study has demonstrated an increase in neutrophil activity in patients who received insulin during the cardiac surgery. The exact mechanism of the increased neutrophil activity is not well understood.[9] Therefore, there are many initiatives in hospitals in the United States focused on achieving control of serum glucose levels after surgical procedures in patients with diabetes, especially in cardiac surgery.

A significant number of studies have been published on glucose control in cardiac surgical patients. The Portland Diabetic Project has demonstrated a significant impact on outcomes in this group of patients. This project is a prospective nonrandomized, observational study of more than 5000 diabetic patients treated between 1987 and 2005.[10] Early on in 1987 these researchers hypothesized that perioperative hyperglycemia contributed to adverse events in cardiac surgical patients and the use of a continuous insulin infusion would eliminate the "incremental risks" that had been attributed to diabetes in this group of patients. Study results demonstrated hyperglycemia during the first 3 postoperative days is predictive of mortality ($P<.0001$), deep sternal wound infection ($P = .0002$), and increased length of stay ($P<.002$). The use of continuous insulin infusions using target blood glucose levels reduced the risk of death (60% reduction) and sternal wound infection (77% reduction). Elevated hemoglobin A1c levels on admission indicated increased risk for sternal wound infections.

The target blood glucose level for their protocol was less than 150 mg/dL maintained for 3 days postoperatively.[10]

Given that 38% of patients admitted to the hospital are diabetics, one can assume the major portion of this group have a history of CVD that may account for the hospital admission. Hyperglycemia is a common finding among medical and surgical patients during hospital admission and estimated to occur in 40% of patients.[11] During the hospital admission, clinicians are challenged to achieve glucose control to prevent adverse events. The subsequent content will focus on intensive insulin therapy for the management of hyperglycemia hospitalized patients in the ICU.

GLUCOSE CONTROL IN THE ICU

Critically ill patients experience stress hyperglycemia. Before 2001, stress hyperglycemia was defined as a blood glucose (BG) level greater than 180 to 200 mg/dL. Some question if this is an adaptive response by the body for the purpose of providing a constant source of fuel to the cells. What is known is stress hyperglycemia (short term and long term) is associated with worse outcomes.[12] The effects of hyperglycemia are such that a BG at 150 mg/dL results in proliferation of white blood cells, activation of proinflammatory cytokines impairing insulin effect in the peripheral tissues, and the onset of insulin resistance. At 180 mg/dL the 3 "P's" occur: polyuria, polydipsia, and polyphagia. It is not uncommon for critically ill patients to have BG levels exceeding 200 mg/dL. This, in addition to the negative outcomes associated with hyperglycemia, triggered several important studies in the last decade for the purpose of identifying a target BG range for critically ill patients.

Two of these studies were conducted in Switzerland and are often referred to as the Leuven Intensive Insulin Therapy (IIT) Trials.[13,14] The first was conducted in a surgical ICU. Patient populations included cardiac and thoracic surgery, multiple trauma, and abdominal and vascular surgery. The investigators demonstrated tight glycemic control using IIT improved the outcome of critically ill surgical patients, resulting in lower mortality rates and a lower incidence of central line blood stream infections (CL-BSIs).[13] Based on this study, tight glycemic control was rapidly adopted as the standard of care using the range of 90 to 120 mg/dL. Van den Berghe's second study was conducted in a medical ICU using the same IIT as previously. In this study, the investigators were able to achieve glucose control but did not see a significant reduction in mortality rates. However, morbidity was reduced with a reduction in acute kidney injury. Patients were weaned from ventilators more quickly and there was a shorter ICU length of stay (LOS). Mortality rates for patients with ICU LOS less than 3 days and receiving intensive insulin therapy were higher.[14] This second study caused many critical care practitioners to rethink tight glucose control.

A few years later the results of another major study were reported. The *N*ormoglycemia in *I*ntensive *C*are *E*valuation—*S*urvival *U*sing *G*lucose *A*lgorithm *R*egulation

(NICE–SUGAR) trial involved 6104 patients in medical and surgical ICUs divided equally between two groups. The control group (3050 patients) had a target BG level of 180 mg/dL or less while the IIT group (3054 patients) had a target BG of 81 to 108 mg/dL. The mortality rate in the control group was 24.9% compared to the mortality rate in the IIT group of 27.5%. The investigators concluded ITT was associated with higher mortality rates.[15] This study led many in critical care to revise their insulin algorithms and protocols to a target glucose range of 140 to 180 mg/dL while some still questioned what the ideal target range should be.

Marik and Preiser conducted a systematic review and meta-analysis for the purpose of identifying all randomized controlled trials (RCTs) comparing mortality of ICU patients randomized to tight glucose control (BG 80–110 mg/dL) compared to patients with less restrictive control. Their outcome criteria included 28-day mortality, need for dialysis, hospital acquired blood stream infections (BSIs), and incidence of hypoglycemia defined as a BG less than 40 mg/dL. Tight glucose control did not reduce 28-day mortality, incidence of BSIs, and requirement for continuous renal replacement therapy. Tight glucose control was associated with a higher incidence of hypoglycemia and increased risk of death in patents not receiving parenteral nutrition.[12] Others have commented on the incidence of hypoglycemia associated with tight glucose control.[16]

Hypoglycemia is not a benign event. Researchers estimate severe hypoglycemia (BG <40 mg/dL) occurs in approximately 18% of patients.[12] Severe hypoglycemia is associated with an increased risk of death. If a patient has two hypoglycemic events within 24 hours of admission to the ICU, risk of death is higher.[17] Patients with traumatic brain injury have an increased risk of brain energy crises and death in the setting of severe hypoglycemia. Hypoglycemia and euglycemia occur at a time when there is increased cerebral metabolic demand but the blood glucose is not adequate. Recognition of this crisis in these patients may be delayed.[17]

Patients at greater risk for hypoglycemia or hyperglycemia include those who may be placed on NPO status; have a change in medications, that is, started on vasopressors or corticosteroids; prolonged use of a regular insulin sliding scale; poor coordination of BG testing and administration of mealtime insulin; and lack of effective communication during patient handoffs from one department to another or one care giver to another.[1] This list is not all inclusive, but represents some of the hazards associated with glucose management.

The current recommendation for serum glucose thresholds for critical care patients is a BG less than 180 mg/dL. Researchers suggest a range of 140 to 180 mg/dL with a possible greater benefit at lower range. Target BG levels less than 110 mg/dL are not recommended at this time.[1] For patients outside of the ICU, the American Diabetes Association (ADA) recommends BG levels 100 to 140 mg/dL, indicating reassessment of the insulin regimen if levels fall below 100 mg/dL to avoid hypoglycemia.[1]

TRANSITIONING FROM INSULIN INFUSIONS

A common practice for glycemia management in acute care has been to discontinue the insulin infusion and start the patient on a subcutaneous regular insulin protocol. Commonly there are point-of-care (POC) glucose checks before each meal and again at bedtime. Regular insulin is administered using a sliding scale based on the glucose result. Studies have shown blood glucose levels to be inadequate after the discontinuation of the insulin infusion, with episodes of hypoglycemia as well as hyperglycemia.[18,19] As a result, many clinicians are changing their practice and prescribing transition protocols to be implemented with the discontinuation of the insulin infusion.

Box 1		
Example: Transitioning insulin from infusion to a basal bolus regimen		
Step 1: Calculate total daily dose (TDD) of insulin by adding amount of insulin infused over previous 4 hours. Multiply × 5.		
Time	**Diabetic Finger Stick**	**Units/mL per Hour**
0300	105	3.2 units
0400	103	3.0 units
0500	91	2.2 units
0600	114	3.8 units
4 hour total		(12.2) 12 units
× 5	TDD	60 units

Step 2: Basal insulin dose to equal 50% of TDD = 30 units.
Step 3: Short-acting insulin to equal 1/3 TDD administered with each meal = 10 units and adjust using sliding scale based on BG obtained before each meal.

Generally, the protocol will be based on calculating the total daily dose (TDD) of insulin based on the amount received during the previous 24 hours. Fifty-percent of the TDD will be administered in the form of a basal insulin. The remaining 50% will be divided into three doses using short-acting insulin to be given at meal times to correct the increased glucose level that is likely to be associated with the meal. The TDD of insulin will be calculated daily based on the total insulin administered the previous day. The basal insulin will be adjusted daily based on the TDD calculation using a sliding scale. The short-acting insulin will be adjusted using a sliding scale not only with the POC testing at each meal but also based on the TDD calculation. Refer to **Box 1** for an example.

This type of protocol is complex and often difficult for health care providers to follow. Care should be taken to simplify the physician order set assuring clarity. The use of a worksheet for the calculations of the TDD and insulin dosing may be helpful. **Box 2** lists some of the challenges associated with the implementation of a transition process.

BLOOD GLUCOSE VARIABILITY

It is not uncommon to see patients having wide swings in their BG levels from levels greater than 200 mg/dL to a sudden drop after insulin administration to 80 or 90 mg/dL and sometimes lower. This variability carries several consequences with it. An obvious result is increased hospital LOS and higher mortality rates. BG variability

Box 2
Challenges associated with implementation of insulin transition protocol
1. Health care provider orders are complex, difficult to follow
2. Education of staff followed by reinforcement
3. Determining the best time to stop the insulin infusion
4. Calculating and planning basal and short-acting insulin doses
5. Shifting from intravenous feeding to oral intake

*Data from*Avanzini F, Marelli G, Donzelli W, et al. Transition from intravenous to subcutaneous insulin. Diabetes Care 2011;34:1445–50.

occurs with tight glucose control and contributes to ICU and hospital mortality at both high and low ranges of blood glucose.[17,20–23] The variability contributes to increased oxidative stress, neuronal and mitochondrial damage, activation of coagulation cascade, and enhancement of cellular apoptosis.[23] It is important for all health care providers to understand the seriousness of this complication.

ISSUES WITH BLOOD GLUCOSE MEASUREMENTS

Blood glucose measurements have been shown to be problematic related to where the blood sample is obtained, and POC device technology including the effects of medications on the device measurement. The following section reviews these considerations.

Sample Site Issues

Blood samples for glucose measurements may be obtained from venous sites, arterial catheters, as well as fingertips. The fingertip sample is similar physiologically to capillary blood. The ADA recommends using venous blood samples because capillary blood sampling may lead to measurement error.[24] Generally arterial blood glucose levels are higher than capillary blood, which are slightly higher than venous blood levels. Differences between capillary and venous glucose levels generally are not significant in normotensive fasting individuals. However, there is the potential for an 8% higher blood glucose level if glucose solutions are changed. In addition, shock states have been found to be associated with increased glucose extraction, causing capillary glucose levels to be lower than those of venous blood. Arterial and central venous blood glucose levels may be underestimated when the clinician obtains a capillary blood glucose sample in a hypotensive patient, which may result in an incorrect diagnosis of hypoglycemia.[24]

POC Devices

Another factor that may affect glucose measurement is the POC device that is used. In the 1970s POC devices were developed to allow for self-monitoring, providing a quick and easy blood glucose measurement. Their success led to these same devices using the same technology being marketed for use in the hospital environment either unchanged or repackaged as a hospital product. Subsequently other devices were developed specifically for hospital use. The use of these is the standard of care across most hospital systems. Certainly they are convenient to use, providing an almost immediate result when compared to the clinical laboratory measurement process. However, their main disadvantage is their lack of accuracy when compared with the central laboratory measurement.[24] The inaccuracy can be attributed to the enzymatic technique used by the POC device. Several studies have shown increased risk for errors based on the type of enzyme used with individual device. Some devices have been shown to underestimate blood glucose levels at increased altitudes, with a 1% to 2% change for every 1000 feet of elevation. Others have shown errors of 15% or greater when analyzing blood in a hypoxic patient with a Pao_2 less than 44 mm Hg.[24]

A secondary consideration is how some medications affect the measurement. Dopamine, acetaminophen, and mannitol have been found to either overestimate or underestimate the glucose level depending on the type of enzyme used when compared to the central laboratory value.[24]

Today, these devices are closely regulated by the U.S. Food and Drug Administration (FDA). Manufacturers are required to demonstrate accuracy of their devices as well as provide supporting evidence of testing for factors contributing to an inaccurate result. Variation in glucose measurements by the central laboratory may vary by 2.2% to 2.8%. However, POC devices may have a greater variation. The FDA assembled a panel in 1996 calling for POC devices to be within 10% total error. Today, the FDA guideline has not changed significantly. The FDA target for accuracy is 95% of readings must be within 20% of the reference for glucose measurements 75 mg/dL or greater and within 15 mg/dL of reference within the hypoglycemic range.[24] For a glucose measurement of 100 mg/dL, this could mean the actual measurement is 80 mg/dL or 120 mg/dL. In spite of this, there is still the potential for problems and serious clinical errors. The FDA also recommends these devices should not be used in critically ill patients.[25] As a safety net, most hospital central laboratories monitor their POC devices closely, following practice guidelines as mandated by their professional certifying organizations as well as requiring the clinical staff to obtain quality control measurements.

NURSING PRACTICE ISSUES

Glucose management falls to the bedside nurse. Insulin administration is managed by the nurse regardless of the route (infusion or subcutaneous). Orders are often complex and difficult to follow. These challenges are reviewed in the following sections.

Implementation of Insulin Protocols

Implementation of an insulin protocol requires extensive education of the nursing staff. The protocols are a paradigm shift for management of glucose levels from use of a regular insulin sliding scale based on every-4-hour POC testing to hourly POC testing and adjustment of the insulin infusion. Also, the protocol may be difficult to read and implement. Several have commented on the importance of educating the staff before the initiation of the protocol and reinforcing the education with the staff once the implementation phase has begun.[18,26-28] There are software-based algorithms available for purchase, which helps with the insulin calculations and have been shown to make it easier for the bedside nurse, that is, fewer mathematical errors and other problems. A limitation of these products is that they are frequently based on one protocol and may not use the algorithm unique to a particular institution.

Management of Insulin Infusions

Insulin infusion protocols often require hourly POC testing to ensure close monitoring of glucose levels. The insulin infusion is often adjusted hourly using a formula based on the result. This process directly impacts the work of the nurse. The nurse must understand and implement the protocol, obtain the blood sample, perform the POC testing, adjust the rate of the infusion, and document the results. Aragon and colleagues conducted an observational and exploratory study for the purpose of evaluating the nursing work incurred and nursing perceptions about tight glycemic control.[27] The investigators reported that although the nurses believed glycemic control was important, the work associated with achieving this goal was substantial. The average time for blood glucose measurements and adjustment of the insulin infusion was 4.72 minutes. If a quality control check is required, the time could be longer. Some facilities require a second nurse to check changes in infusion rates, which can contribute to increased nursing time. This could require up to 2 hours in a 24-hour period for glucose control for one patient.[27] In this study, the estimated costs of the time spent on glucose control during a 1-year period were $182,488 for nursing salaries and $58,000 in supply costs.[27] Others have commented on the increased nursing labor.[26] Often critical care nurses can be heard requesting continuous blood glucose technology be implemented at the bedside.

Continuous Blood Glucose Measurements

A minimum blood glucose sampling rate of one value every 4 hours does not exclude that peak or trough values in between two measurements could have been missed, which could have had an influence on the calculated indices.[22] Probably only a continuous blood glucose sensor would be able to offer the optimal sampling rate. Development of continuous blood glucose technology for use at the bedside is in the developmental/validation stage by several companies. Their greatest challenge is obtaining tight correlation with the laboratory measurement. In the best of circumstances, a closed loop system would be ideal. However, just having a continuous blood glucose measurement available would ideally avoid some of the fluctuations currently seen leading to a more consistent level and save the nurse time.

SUMMARY

Inpatient glucose control today is complex and challenging for the clinician. The importance of avoiding wide swings in the BG levels and hypoglycemic events cannot be underestimated. Nurses must be at the table as insulin protocols or physician order sets are being developed to address issues with readability and understanding. Education of all staff is extremely important with follow-up education at intervals for both nurses and physician providers. While there are no official guidelines for quality of inpatient glycemic control, a multidisciplinary team consisting of key physicians (endocrinology and others), clinical nurse specialists, and diabetes educator and clinical pharmacist can develop quality improvement projects for monitoring and process improvement.[29] Continuous monitoring of practices will reduce the risk for errors and support safe practices.

REFERENCES

1. Moghissi ES, Korytkowski MT, DiNardo M, et al. American Association of Clinical Endocrinologists and American Diabetes Association Consensus Statement on Inpatient Glycemic Control. Endocr Pract 2009;15(4):1–17.
2. Umpierrez GE, Isaacs, Bazargan N, et al. Hyperglycemia: an independent marker of in-hospital mortality in patients with undiagnosed diabetes. J Clin Endocrinol Metab 2002;87:978–82.
3. Stentz FB, Umpierrez GE, Cuervo R, et al. Proinflammatory cytokines, markers of cardiovascular risks, oxidative stress, and lipid peroxidation in patients with hyperglycemic crises. Diabetes 2004;53:2079–86.
4. Read JL, Cheng EY. Intensive insulin therapy for acute hyperglycemia. AACN Adv Crit Care 2007;18(2):200–12.
5. Krinsley JS, Jones RL. Cost analysis of intensive glycemic control in critically ill patients. Chest 2006;129:644–50.
6. Van den Berghe G, Wouters PJ, Kesteloot K, et al. Analysis of healthcare resource utilization in intensive insulin therapy in critically ill patients. Crit Care Med 2006;34(3):612–6.
7. Mazzone T. Intensive glucose lowering and cardiovascular disease prevention in diabetes: reconciling the recent clinical trial data. Circulation 2010;122:2201–11.
8. Ata A, Lee J, Bestle SL, et al. Postoperative hyperglycemia and surgical site infection in general surgery patients. Arch Surg 2010;145(9):858–64.

9. Rassia AJ, Givan AL, Marrin AS, et al. Insulin increases neutrophils count and phagocytic activity after cardiac surgery. Anesth Analg 2002;94:1113–9.
10. Furnary AP, Wu YX. Clinical effects of hyperglycemia in the cardiac surgery population: The Portland Diabetic Project. Endocrinol Pract 2006;12(Suppl 3):22–6.
11. Qaseem A, Humphrey LL, Chou R, et al. Use of intensive insulin therapy for the management of glycemic control in hospitalized patients: a clinical practice guideline from the American College of Physicians. Ann Intern Med 2011;154:260–7.
12. Marik PE, Preiser JC. Toward understanding tight glycemic control in the ICU: a systematic review and metanalysis. Chest 2010;137(3):544–51.
13. Van den Berghe G, Wouters P, Weekers F, et al. Intensive insulin therapy in critically ill patients. N Engl J Med 2001;345(19):1359–67.
14. Van den Berghe G, Wilmer A, Hermans G, et al. Intensive insulin therapy in the medical ICU. N Engl J Med 2006;354(5):449–61.
15. NICE-SUGAR Investigators, Finfer S, Chittock DR, Su SY, et al.Intensive versus conventional glucose control in critically ill patients. N Engl J Med 2009;360(13): 1283–97.
16. Wiener RS, Wiener DC, Larson RJ. Benefits and risks of tight glucose control in critically ill adults. JAMA 2008;300(8):933–44.
17. Bagshaw SM, Bellomo R, Jacka MJ, et al. The impact of early hypoglycemia and blood glucose variability on outcome of critical illness. Crit Care 2009;13:R91.
18. Avanzini F, Marelli G, Donzelli W, et al. Transition from intravenous to subcutaneous insulin. Diabetes Care 2011;34:1445–50.
19. Weant KA, Ladha A. Conversion from continuous insulin infusions to subcutaneous insulin in critically ill patients. Ann Pharmacother 2009;43:629–34.
20. Krinsley JS. Glycemic variability and mortality in critically ill patients: the impact of diabetes. J Diabetes Technol 2009;3(6):1292–1301.
21. Krinsley JS. Editorials: Glycemic variability in critical illness and the end of chapter 1. Crit Care Med 2010;38(4):1207.
22. Meyfroidt G, Keenan DM, Wang X, et al. Dynamic characteristics of blood glucose time series during the course of critical illness: effects of intensive insulin therapy and relative association with mortality. Crit Care Med 2010;38(4):1021–9.
23. Hermandides J, Vriesendorp TM, Bosman RJ, et al. Glucose variability is associated with intensive care unit mortality. Crit Care Med 2010;38(3):838–42.
24. Rice MJ, Pitkin AD, Coursin DB. Glucose measurement in the operating room: More complicated than it seems. Anesth Analg 2010;110(4):1056–65.
25. Fahy BG, Sheehy AM, Coursin DB. Glucose control in the intensive care unit. Crit Care Med 2009;37:1769–76.
26. Eigsti, E, Henke K. Innovative solutions: development and implementation of a tight blood glucose management protocol. Dimens Crit Care Nurs 2006;25(2):62–5.
27. Aragon D. Evaluation of nursing work effort and perceptions about blood glucose testing in tight glycemic control. Am J Crit Care 2006;15:370–7.
28. Corbin AE, Carmical D, Goetz JA, et al. One institution's experience with implementing protocols for glycemic management. Dimens Crit Care Nurs 2010;29(4):167–72.
29. Schnipper JL, Magee M, Larsen K, et al. Society of Hospital Medicine Glycemic Control Task Force Summary: practice recommendations for assessing the impact of glycemic control efforts. J Hosp Med 2008;3(5 Suppl 5):S66–S75.

Index

Note: Page numbers of article titles are in **boldface** type.

D

United States Postal Service

Statement of Ownership, Management, and Circulation
(All Periodicals Publications Except Requestor Publications)

1. Publication Title	2. Publication Number	3. Filing Date
Critical Care Nursing Clinics of North America	0 0 6 - 2 7 3	9/16/11

4. Issue Frequency	5. Number of Issues Published Annually	6. Annual Subscription Price
Mar, Jun, Sep, Dec	4	$135.00

7. Complete Mailing Address of Known Office of Publication (Not printer) (Street, city, county, state, and ZIP+4®)

Elsevier Inc.
360 Park Avenue South
New York, NY 10010-1710

Contact Person
Amy S. Beacham

Telephone (Include area code)
215-239-3687

8. Complete Mailing Address of Headquarters or General Business Office of Publisher (Not printer)

Elsevier Inc., 360 Park Avenue South, New York, NY 10010-1710

9. Full Names and Complete Mailing Addresses of Publisher, Editor, and Managing Editor (Do not leave blank)

Publisher (Name and complete mailing address)

Kim Murphy, Elsevier, Inc., 1600 John F. Kennedy Blvd. Suite 1800, Philadelphia, PA 19103-2899

Editor (Name and complete mailing address)

Katie Hartner, Elsevier, Inc., 1600 John F. Kennedy Blvd. Suite 1800, Philadelphia, PA 19103-2899

Managing Editor (Name and complete mailing address)

Sarah Barth, Elsevier, Inc., 1600 John F. Kennedy Blvd. Suite 1800, Philadelphia, PA 19103-2899

10. Owner (Do not leave blank. If the publication is owned by a corporation, give the name and address of the corporation immediately followed by the names and addresses of all stockholders owning or holding 1 percent or more of the total amount of stock. If not owned by a corporation, give the names and addresses of the individual owners. If owned by a partnership or other unincorporated firm, give its name and address as well as those of each individual owner. If the publication is published by a nonprofit organization, give its name and address.)

Full Name	Complete Mailing Address
Wholly owned subsidiary of	4520 East-West Highway
Reed/Elsevier, US holdings	Bethesda, MD 20814

11. Known Bondholders, Mortgagees, and Other Security Holders Owning or Holding 1 Percent or More of Total Amount of Bonds, Mortgages, or Other Securities. If none, check box ☐ None

Full Name	Complete Mailing Address
N/A	

12. Tax Status (For completion by nonprofit organizations authorized to mail at nonprofit rates) (Check one)
The purpose, function, and nonprofit status of this organization and the exempt status for federal income tax purposes:
☐ Has Not Changed During Preceding 12 Months
☐ Has Changed During Preceding 12 Months (Publisher must submit explanation of change with this statement)

13. Publication Title	14. Issue Date for Circulation Data Below
Critical Care Nursing Clinics of North America	June 2011

15. Extent and Nature of Circulation			Average No. Copies Each Issue During Preceding 12 Months	No. Copies of Single Issue Published Nearest to Filing Date
a. Total Number of Copies (Net press run)			941	920
b. Paid Circulation (By Mail and Outside the Mail)	(1)	Mailed Outside-County Paid Subscriptions Stated on PS Form 3541 (Include paid distribution above nominal rate, advertiser's proof copies, and exchange copies)	502	444
	(2)	Mailed In-County Paid Subscriptions Stated on PS Form 3541 (Include paid distribution above nominal rate, advertiser's proof copies, and exchange copies)		
	(3)	Paid Distribution Outside the Mails Including Sales Through Dealers and Carriers, Street Vendors, Counter Sales, and Other Paid Distribution Outside USPS®	102	88
	(4)	Paid Distribution by Other Classes Mailed Through the USPS (e.g. First-Class Mail®)		
c. Total Paid Distribution (Sum of 15b (1), (2), (3), and (4))	►		604	532
d. Free or Nominal Rate Distribution (By Mail and Outside the Mail)	(1)	Free or Nominal Rate Outside-County Copies Included on PS Form 3541	60	51
	(2)	Free or Nominal Rate In-County Copies Included on PS Form 3541		
	(3)	Free or Nominal Rate Copies Mailed at Other Classes Through the USPS (e.g. First-Class Mail)		
	(4)	Free or Nominal Rate Distribution Outside the Mail (Carriers or other means)		
e. Total Free or Nominal Rate Distribution (Sum of 15d (1), (2), (3) and (4))	►		60	51
f. Total Distribution (Sum of 15c and 15e)	►		664	583
g. Copies not Distributed (See instructions to publishers #4 (page #3))	►		277	337
h. Total (Sum of 15f and g)	►		941	920
i. Percent Paid (15c divided by 15f times 100)			90.96%	91.25%

16. Publication of Statement of Ownership

☐ If the publication is a general publication, publication of this statement is required. Will be printed ☐ Publication not required in the December 2011 issue of this publication.

17. Signature and Title of Editor, Publisher, Business Manager, or Owner

[signature] Amy S. Beacham – Senior Inventory Distribution Coordinator

Date: September 16, 2011

I certify that all information furnished on this form is true and complete. I understand that anyone who furnishes false or misleading information on this form or who omits material or information requested on the form may be subject to criminal sanctions (including fines and imprisonment) and/or civil sanctions (including civil penalties).

PS Form **3526**, September 2007 (Page 2 of 3)

PS Form **3526**, September 2007 (Page 1 of 3) (Instructions Page 3)   PSN 7530-01-000-9931 **PRIVACY NOTICE**: See our Privacy policy in www.usps.com

Moving?

Make sure your subscription moves with you!

To notify us of your new address, find your **Clinics Account Number** (located on your mailing label above your name), and contact customer service at:

Email: journalscustomerservice-usa@elsevier.com

800-654-2452 (subscribers in the U.S. & Canada)
314-447-8871 (subscribers outside of the U.S. & Canada)

Fax number: 314-447-8029

Elsevier Health Sciences Division
Subscription Customer Service
3251 Riverport Lane
Maryland Heights, MO 63043

*To ensure uninterrupted delivery of your subscription, please notify us at least 4 weeks in advance of move.

Printed and bound by CPI Group (UK) Ltd, Croydon, CR0 4YY

13/10/2024

01773590-0002